T0259442

Foot and Ankle Trauma

Guest Editor

DENISE M. MANDI, DPM

CLINICS IN PODIATRIC MEDICINE AND SURGERY

www.podiatric.theclinics.com

Consulting Editor
THOMAS ZGONIS, DPM, FACFAS

April 2012 • Volume 29 • Number 2

SAUNDERS an imprint of ELSEVIER, Inc.

W.B. SAUNDERS COMPANY
A Division of Elsevier Inc.

1600 John F. Kennedy Boulevard ● Suite 1800 ● Philadelphia, Pennsylvania 19103-2899

http://www.theclinics.com

CLINICS IN PODIATRIC MEDICINE AND SURGERY Volume 29, Number 2
April 2012 ISSN 0891-8422, ISBN-13: 978-1-4557-3922-6

Editor: Patrick Manley

Clinics in Podiatric Medicine and Surgery (ISSN 0891-8422) is published quarterly by Elsevier Inc., 360 Park Avenue South, New York, NY 10010-1710. Months of issue are January, April, July, and October. Business and Editorial Offices: 1600 John F. Kennedy Blvd., Ste. 1800, Philadelphia, PA 19103-2899. Customer Service Office: 3251 Riverport Lane, Maryland Heights, MO 63043. Periodicals postage paid at New York, NY and additional mailing offices. Subscription prices are $292.00 per year for US individuals, $410.00 per year for US institutions, $148.00 per year for US students and residents, $350.00 per year for Canadian individuals, $508.00 for Canadian institutions, $415.00 for international individuals, $508.00 per year for international institutions and $208.00 per year for Canadian and foreign students/residents. To receive student/resident rate, orders must be accompanied by name of affiliated institution, date of term, and the *signature* of program/residency coordinator on institution letterhead. Orders will be billed at individual rate until proof of status is received. Foreign air speed delivery is included in all *Clinics* subscription prices. All prices are subject to change without notice. POSTMASTER: Send address changes to *Clinics in Podiatric Medicine and Surgery*, Elsevier Health Sciences Division, Subscription Customer Service, 3251 Riverport Lane, Maryland Heights, MO 63043. **Customer Service: 1-800-654-2452 (US). From outside of the US, call 314-447-8871. Fax: 314-447-8029. E-mail: JournalsCustomerService-usa@elsevier.com (for print support); JournalsOnlineSupport-usa@elsevier.com (for online support).**

Reprints. For copies of 100 or more of articles in this publication, please contact the Commercial Reprints Department, Elsevier Inc., 360 Park Avenue South, New York, NY 10010-1710. Tel.: 212-633-3812; Fax: 212-462-1935; E-mail: reprints@elsevier.com.

Clinics in Podiatric Medicine and Surgery is covered in *MEDLINE/PubMed (Index Medicus)* and *EMBASE/Excerpta Medica*.

Printed and bound by CPI Group (UK) Ltd, Croydon, CR0 4YY

Transferred to Digital Print 2012

Contributors

CONSULTING EDITOR

THOMAS ZGONIS, DPM, FACFAS
Associate Professor, Reconstructive Foot and Ankle Fellowship Director and Chief,
Division of Podiatric Medicine and Surgery, Department of Orthopedic Surgery,
The University of Texas Health Science Center at San Antonio, San Antonio, Texas

GUEST EDITOR

DENISE M. MANDI, DPM
Section Chief, Foot & Ankle Surgery, Department of Surgery, Broadlawns Medical Center,
Des Moines, Iowa

AUTHORS

JUSTIN BANKS
Third Year Medical Student, Des Moines University, Des Moines, Iowa

BRANDON BARRETT
Third Year Medical Student, Des Moines University, Des Moines, Iowa

RON P. BELIN, DPM
Trauma Fellow, Section of Foot & Ankle Surgery, Department of Surgery, Broadlawns
Medical Center, Des Moines, Iowa

NICHOLAS J. BEVILACQUA, DPM, FACFAS
North Jersey Orthopaedic Specialists, Teaneck, North Jersey

DAVI CROSS, DPM
Resident, Heritage Valley Health System, Beaver, Pennsylvania

LAWRENCE A. DIDOMENICO, DPM, FACFAS
Director of Reconstructive Rearfoot and Ankle Surgical Fellowship, Section Director-St.
Elizabeth Hospital, Youngstown; Adjunct Professor, Ohio College of Podiatric Medicine,
Independence, Ohio

BRENT D. HAVERSTOCK, DPM, FACFAS
Chief, Section of Podiatric Surgery, Clinical Assistant Professor of Surgery, University
of Calgary, Faculty of Medicine, Peter Lougheed Centre, Calgary, Alberta, Canada

BLAKE HINES, BA
Third Year DPM Student, Des Moines University, Des Moines, Iowa

NICOLE JEDLICKA, DPM
Covenant Medical Center, Waterloo, Iowa

DENISE M. MANDI, DPM
Section Chief, Foot & Ankle Surgery, Department of Surgery, Broadlawns Medical Center, Des Moines, Iowa

MICA M. MURDOCH, DPM, FACFAS
Broadlawns Medical Center, Des Moines, Iowa

MICHAEL MURDOCK, DPM
Covenant Medical Center, Waterloo, Iowa

BEN L. OLSEN, DPM, FACFAS
Director, Foot and Ankle Trauma Fellowship, Department of Foot and Ankle Surgery, Broadlawns Medical Center, Des Moines, Iowa

KATHIE PALMERSHEIM, BS
Third Year DPM Student, Des Moines University, Des Moines, Iowa

CRYSTAL L. RAMANUJAM, DPM, MSc
Assistant Professor, Division of Podiatric Medicine and Surgery, Department of Orthopaedic Surgery, University of Texas Health Science Center at San Antonio, San Antonio, Texas

JOHN J. STAPLETON, DPM, FACFAS
Foot and Ankle Surgery, VSAS Orthopaedics; Chief of Podiatric Surgery, Lehigh Valley Hospital, Allentown; Clinical Assistant Professor of Surgery, Penn State College of Medicine, Hershey, Pennsylvania

N. JAKE SUMMERS, BS
College of Podiatric Medicine and Surgery, Des Moines University, Des Moines, Iowa

THOMAS ZGONIS, DPM, FACFAS
Associate Professor, Reconstructive Foot and Ankle Fellowship Director and Chief, Division of Podiatric Medicine and Surgery, Department of Orthopedic Surgery, The University of Texas Health Science Center at San Antonio, San Antonio, Texas

Contents

Foreword: Foot and Ankle Trauma   xi

Thomas Zgonis

Preface: Foot and Ankle Trauma   xiii

Denise M. Mandi

Ankle Fractures   155

Denise M. Mandi

> Ankle fractures are important injuries involving a weight-bearing joint critical to mobility. This article will discuss the necessity of and justification for surgical correction of virtually all ankle fractures. Various ankle fracture types will be explored, mechanisms illuminated and proper treatment outlined for these complex injuries.

Fractures of the Talus: A Comprehensive Review   187

N. Jake Summers and Mica M. Murdoch

> The talus, a highly specialized bone with a unique anatomic design, is crucial for normal ambulation. Although uncommon, talar fractures can be potentially devastating to the patient. Although all talar fractures require appropriate diagnosis and treatment, some require surgical skill for appropriate correction. This article reviews the literature on talar fractures and their treatments.

Calcaneal Fractures: Update on Current Treatments   205

Kathie Palmersheim, Blake Hines, and Ben L. Olsen

> Calcaneal fractures represent 2% of all fractures and account for approximately 60% of all tarsal injuries. Motor vehicle collisions and falls are the major causes of these large force compression injuries, causing widening of the heel, loss of heel height, and articular surface displacement. A correlation has been shown between restoration of normal anatomy and satisfactory functional outcome. Once the basic principles of calcaneal fractures are understood, including the anatomy, the radiographic findings, and the challenges that these complicated fractures present, the physician can then be ready with the armamentarium that allows for a patient-specific and injury-specific plan.

Tarsometatarsal/Lisfranc Joint   221

Lawrence A. DiDomenico and Davi Cross

> Accurate early diagnosis with adequate reduction and maintenance of anatomic alignment of the dislocation or fracture within the Lisfranc joint complex have been found to be the key to successful outcomes regarding this injury. Because of the anatomic variations, the thin soft tissue envelop, and the abundance of ligamentous and capsular structures in the region,

repair of these injuries can be a challenge. The classification systems used to describe these injuries aid in describing the mechanism of injury or displacement type present, which may aid in determining what treatment modality can provide the best outcome.

Pilon Fractures   243

Denise M. Mandi, Ron P. Belin, Justin Banks, and Brandon Barrett

The nature of the pilon fracture has caused evolution of treatment methods and its historically high rate of complication and poor outcome continue to direct choice of treatment. Attention to the delicate soft tissue envelope surrounding the ankle and recognition of the severity of the initial injury is crucial to ensure a satisfactory outcome and to minimize complications. Understanding the importance of staging surgical interventions will help to improve outcomes, but even optimal treatment may result in less than satisfactory results.

Overview of Concepts and Treatments in Open Fractures   279

Nicole Jedlicka, N. Jake Summers, and Mica M. Murdoch

Open fractures are one of the few lower extremity surgical emergencies. These injuries require immediate treatment. If untreated, severe cases of open fracture can be limb threatening. This article is a review of the literature of open fractures and the current treatment guidelines.

Treatment of the Neglected Achilles Tendon Rupture   291

Nicholas J. Bevilacqua

Achilles tendon ruptures are best managed acutely. Neglected Achilles tendon ruptures are debilitating injuries and the increased complexity of the situation must be appreciated. Surgical management is recommended, and only in the poorest surgical candidate is conservative treatment entertained. Numerous treatment algorithms and surgical techniques have been described. A V-Y advancement flap and flexor halluces longus tendon transfer have been found to be reliable and achieve good clinical outcomes for defects ranging from 2 cm to 8 cm. This article focuses on the treatment options for the neglected Achilles tendon rupture.

Compartment Syndrome: A Review of the Literature   301

Michael Murdock and Mica M. Murdoch

Compartment syndrome is a rare but severe complication of lower extremity trauma. This article provides an extensive review of the literature, including incidence, physical examination findings, pathophysiology, compartment pressure evaluation, and surgical decompression techniques. Most of the recent compartment syndrome literature shows case reports of atypical causes of this limb-threatening disorder. Although the emphasis of this article is traumatic compartment syndrome, recent literature on chronic lower extremity compartment syndrome, secondary to exercise or activity, is also discussed.

Puncture Wounds of the Foot   311

Brent D. Haverstock

Puncture wounds often appear benign but can cause significant pedal morbidity. Podiatric physicians who treat such wounds should educate local emergency room, urgent care center, and primary care physicians as to the potential complications associated with puncture wounds. Timely referral, recognition of the potential complications, and appropriate treatment ensure that the wound does not advance beyond a puncture wound. If complications have developed, aggressive treatment is required to eradicate the infection and prevent pedal amputation.

Current Concepts and Techniques in Foot and Ankle Surgery

Versatility of Intrinsic Muscle Flaps for the Diabetic Charcot Foot   323

Crystal L. Ramanujam and Thomas Zgonis

Bone, joint, and/or tendon exposure following surgical debridement of diabetic foot infections requires careful consideration when choosing appropriate closure methods. The unique architecture of the foot, coupled with the functional demands of mobilization, makes soft tissue reconstruction for plantar defects especially challenging. Muscle flaps incorporate the muscle, associated nerve, and vascular pedicles during transposition. This article covers their unique properties for soft tissue coverage in the diabetic Charcot foot.

Total Extrusion of the Cuboid: A Case Report   327

John J. Stapleton

The incidence of total extrusion of the cuboid is rare, without any known published data or surgical guidelines. This case report describes the management of an open extruded cuboid by staged surgical interventions. Arthrodesis of the lateral column with a structural bone graft is a viable option to address the shortening, instability, and severe bone loss caused by the total cuboid extrusion.

Index   331

FORTHCOMING ISSUES

July 2012
Contemporary Controversies in Foot and Ankle Surgery
Neal Blitz, DPM, *Guest Editor*

October 2012
Ankle Arthritis
Jesse B. Burks, DPM, *Guest Editor*

January 2013
Primary Total Ankle Replacement
Thomas S. Roukis, DPM, *Guest Editor*

RECENT ISSUES

January 2012
Arthrodesis of the Foot and Ankle
Steven F. Boc, DPM and
Vincent Muscarella, DPM,
Guest Editors

October 2011
Advances in Fixation Technology for the Foot and Ankle
Patrick R. Burns, DPM, *Guest Editor*

July 2011
Foot and Ankle Arthroscopy
Laurence G. Rubin, DPM, FACFAS,
Guest Editor

THE CLINICS ARE NOW AVAILABLE ONLINE!

Access your subscription at:
www.theclinics.com

Foreword

Foot and Ankle Trauma

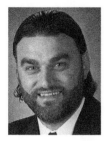

Thomas Zgonis, DPM
Consulting Editor

This issue of *Clinics in Podiatric Medicine and Surgery* brings together experts in the field of foot and ankle trauma to provide us with the most current treatments and fixation methods available for the management of the traumatic patient. Trauma as it relates to the foot and ankle can range from commonly encountered low-energy fractures to severely deformed and mutilated injuries that can be quite challenging before deciding on an effective treatment plan. Throughout this issue, numerous fractures such as the talus, calcaneus, pilon, and Lisfranc's injuries are reviewed in detail. In addition, the management of crush injuries and traumatized soft tissue envelope is also discussed in detail. Postoperative algorithms are presented for the treatment of posttraumatic deformities and/or complications.

Despite the numerous advances in the field of foot and ankle trauma, the realistic outcome for certain select injuries may not quite meet the patient's and surgeon's expectations. Family counseling and education about the severity and prolonged rehabilitation of the patient's injury are paramount for the patient's successful recovery. The guest editor, Dr Denise Mandi, has done an outstanding job with her contributions and invited authors and I thank them for their input in managing these complex foot and ankle injuries.

Thomas Zgonis, DPM
Division of Podiatric Medicine and Surgery
Department of Orthopaedic Surgery
The University of Texas Health Science Center at San Antonio
7703 Floyd Curl Drive–MSC 7776
San Antonio, TX 78229, USA

E-mail address:
zgonis@uthscsa.edu

Clin Podiatr Med Surg 29 (2012) xi
doi:10.1016/j.cpm.2012.02.004 **podiatric.theclinics.com**
0891-8422/12/$ – see front matter © 2012 Elsevier Inc. All rights reserved.

Preface

Foot and Ankle Trauma

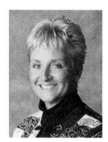

Denise M. Mandi, DPM
Guest Editor

Information is not knowledge. The only source of knowledge is experience.
— *Albert Einstein*

Podiatry has always been proven to be the leader in diagnosing and treating lower extremity pathology, but our prowess at managing foot and ankle trauma is a relatively recent development. Better education and postgraduate training programs focusing on trauma, coupled with physician shortages and increasing patient loads, have opened a door for us to become the preeminent lower extremity trauma experts.

In this issue of the *Clinics in Podiatric Medicine and Surgery*, many busy lower extremity trauma surgeons demonstrate this shift by sharing their knowledge and experience with us. I appreciate the opportunity that Dr Zgonis has given me to be involved with this journal. It has been a privilege to work with these talented individuals and bring you updates on lower extremity trauma and its treatment. Parity for our profession with the rest of medicine will not be achieved through legislation alone, but by the competent and skillful treatment of the pathology that is presented to us. Use the knowledge that is presented here, build your experience, and we can all achieve parity through action.

Denise M. Mandi, DPM
Section of Foot & Ankle Surgery
Department of Surgery
Broadlawns Medical Center
1801 Hickman Road
Des Moines, IA 50314, USA

E-mail address:
dmandi@broadlawns.org

Clin Podiatr Med Surg 29 (2012) xiii
doi:10.1016/j.cpm.2012.02.005
0891-8422/12/$ – see front matter © 2012 Elsevier Inc. All rights reserved.

Ankle Fractures

Denise M. Mandi, DPM

KEYWORDS

- Ankle fractures • Ankle joint • Fibular fracture
- Medial malleolar fracture

All lower extremity surgeons are familiar with the anatomy and biomechanics of the ankle joint, and there is a wealth of information available about the various classification systems for ankle fractures, so these are briefly reviewed in this article. Salient points about the diagnosis and treatment of ankle fractures are shared. Some hypotheses and research findings are proposed to explain phenomena that are familiar in treating these injuries.

After reading this article, readers will understand why these injuries are so significant in practices and in health care at large, will understand the reasoning and justification for the chosen treatments, and will be equipped with the knowledge and understanding necessary to treat these injuries with expertise.

OVERVIEW

Ankle injuries, of all types, are responsible for more than 5 million emergency department visits annually.[1,2] In 2009, the most common lower extremity diagnosis for an emergency department visit in the United States was strain or sprain, at 36% of lower extremity injuries. The average cost of one of those visits was approximately $2000, for a total average annual cost of $10 billion or more for ankle injuries in the United States. A study by Daly and colleagues[3] showed an incidence of ankle fractures of 187 per every 100,000 people per year. Ankle sprains account for 85% of these ankle injuries, with fractures making up the remaining 15% of ankle injuries.[4] Ankle fracture is the most common intra-articular fracture of a weight-bearing joint,[5] and ankle fractures make up 9% of all fractures. The average age of patients with ankle fractures is 46 years, with women slightly more likely affected, at 53%. The most common cause is falls at 37.5%, followed by inversion injuries at 31.5% and sport-related injuries at 10.2% of all ankle fractures.[6]

Of the estimated 585,000 ankle fractures that occur each year in the United States, 25% undergo surgical intervention.[7] The typical cost to treat an ankle sprain or fracture conservatively ranges from $500 to $4000. The cost of surgical treatment can vary from $11,000 to $25,000. Most ankle fractures are isolated injuries. When associated fractures are present, in approximately 5% of patients, they usually affect the

Section of Foot & Ankle Surgery, Department of Surgery, Broadlawns Medical Center, 1801 Hickman Road, Des Moines, IA 50314, USA
E-mail address: dmandi@broadlawns.org

Clin Podiatr Med Surg 29 (2012) 155–186
doi:10.1016/j.cpm.2012.01.002
0891-8422/12/$ – see front matter © 2012 Elsevier Inc. All rights reserved.

podiatric.theclinics.com

ipsilateral lower limb.[8] Recent studies of polytrauma patients, with and without foot and ankle injuries, found that of those who survived their initial injuries, those with foot and ankle fractures had much more functional impairment.[9] We do not perform this surgery just for the thrill of it or to get patients bearing weight faster but to prevent the development of arthritis in the joint. There are data that should be at surgeons' ready to convey the justification for this treatment choice to the patient.

Pott[10] was among the first to stress anatomic reduction in the treatment of ankle fractures, in 1768. Lane[11,12] in 1894 first recommended surgery to achieve anatomic reduction of the ankle, but surgery was reserved for those cases in which closed reduction had been attempted and failed, even though surgical results were less than satisfactory.[13–19] At the time, the medial side of the joint was the focus of the attention, because it was believed that it was necessary to provide a stable pillar for the lower leg.[18,20–26] It was not until 1958, when the Arbeitsgemeinschaft für Osteosynthesefragen [Association for the Study of Internal Fixation] (AO) Group began their study of fracture treatment, that the previous work of Lane, Danis,[27] and other likeminded physicians slowly became appreciated and expanded.[28,29] Several biomechanical, anatomic, and clinical studies in the 1970s showed the importance of precise anatomic reduction of the medial and lateral malleoli in ankle fractures and suddenly excellent results were found.[30–36] In 1998, Carr and Trafton[37] stated, "The quality of the reduction is more important than whether it was achieved by open or closed techniques." They also believed that although closed reduction restores the tibiotalar relationship, it rarely reduces the lateral malleolus to its anatomic position due to the residual shortening or rotation that occurs.[38]

The ankle joint is essential to maintaining upright posture and to ambulation. The ankle joint is a complex hinge-type joint, similar to the mortise and tenon joint of carpentry. The stability of the ankle joint is maintained by a combination of its bony architecture and the surrounding musculature and ligamentous structures.[39,40] The ankle has the smallest surface area of the major weight-bearing joints. Ambulation produces stresses across the ankle joint anywhere from 1.25 to 5.5 times normal body weight, depending on activity, which is more than twice the force found in the hip or knee.[37] The small size and large stresses across the ankle set up a situation there are many pounds per square inch of pressure across its articular cartilage. Combined with a complex combination of motion occurring at or near the ankle joint, it is easy to understand why there is much ankle pain in practices. In 1931, Bohler[41] stated, "the joints that are no longer congruent are therefore abraded. With time, the greater the displacement, the more pronounced the arthritic changes. The ankle joint remains permanently painful."

The talar dome bears more weight per unit area than any other joint surface. The ankle is sensitive to even small tibiotalar incongruency.[42] As Yablon and colleagues[42] stated, in bimalleolar ankle fractures, "the talus faithfully followed...the lateral malleolus," causing derangement of the contact between the tibia and talus. In their research at the Alfred I. duPont Institute, Ramsey and Hamilton[34] presented perhaps the most important indication for surgical treatment of ankle fractures. Previous studies had shown that long-term results of ankle injuries, where residual talar displacement was noted, had unsatisfactory results.[30,43,44] Ramsey and Hamilton[34] postulated, "the area of contact between the articular surfaces of the tibiotalar joint is altered and may contribute to the poor result." Their research results showed that a 1-mm lateral shift of the talus produced a 42% reduction in tibiotalar contact area. Zindrick and coworkers[45] added, in 1985, that this loss of contact area concentrated the stress across the articular surface, causing a 49% increase in the joint contact pressure.

So, with a mere 1 mm of lateral displacement of the talus, the combination of decreased surface area and increased contact pressures across the ankle joint articular cartilage, if left unaddressed, results in cartilage wear and arthritis. A lateral shift of 2 mm or more of the talus is generally considered an indication for surgical treatment,[5,43,46–49] as is 2 mm to 3 mm of displacement of either malleolus. These findings opens virtually all ankle fractures to surgical reduction, but additional research and clinical results may refute this in some cases. Furthermore, the author recommends postponing surgical intervention of most closed fractures for 1 to 2 weeks due to soft tissue considerations (discussed later). **Table 1** shows results comparing nonoperative and surgical management of ankle fractures using AO Group principles, illustrating the importance of accurate anatomic reduction in displaced fractures.[6]

For ease and consistency, fractures using a combination of the Henderson descriptive classification systems and the Danis-Weber (D-W) classification system are discussed.[50,51] Although D-W does not include medial side injury, combining it with Henderson's bimalleolar and trimalleolar descriptions provides a comprehensive and simple system. D-W type A represents a fibular fracture distal to the joint, type B represents a fibular fracture at the level of the joint, and type C a fibular fracture proximal to joint level.[29,52,53] D-W fracture types by prevalence are type A—29.7%, type B—62.5%, and type C—7.8%.[54] Proximal fibular/Maisonneuve fractures, open fractures, and complications are also discussed (**Figs. 1–3**).

Unlike many colleagues, the author does not use the Lauge-Hansen classification system. Although it is a comprehensive classification system, it is cumbersome. Because it is based on cadaver study, it represents some fractures not often seen clinically. Also, in the author's opinion, a good classification system should be easy to use and should clearly direct treatment, and the Lauge-Hansen system often falls short on both points. I believe that the AO Group classification system, although not widely adopted by podiatry, is the best currently in use.

OVERVIEW OF ISOLATED FIBULAR FRACTURES

Lateral malleolar fractures tend to affect an older patient population after low-energy trauma, whereas medial malleolar fractures tend to occur in younger patients after high-energy trauma[6]; 70% of all D-W types A and B fractures are isolated lateral malleolar fractures, 6.3% are isolated medial malleolar fractures, 16% are bimalleolar fractures, and 7.5% trimalleolar.[54] Although the fibula bears little body weight, its importance as gatekeeper of the ankle architecture is immense. Many investigators believe, as does the author, that in ankle fractures, the distal fibular fracture is the dominant fracture and commands attention if satisfactory results are to be achieved.[38] In 1979, Thordarson and colleagues[55] studied the effects of fibular shortening, lateral

Table 1
Effect of reduction quality and fracture type on post-injury pain and development of osteoarthritis (OA)

Danis-Weber Type	A	B	C
Adequate reduction	0% Rearfoot pain 0% OA	23% Rearfoot pain 0% OA	20% Rearfoot pain 20% OA
Inadequate reduction	50% Rearfoot pain 100% OA	64% Rearfoot pain 90% OA	69% Rearfoot pain 100% OA
Surgical reduction	81% Good–excellent	81% Good–excellent	72% Good–excellent

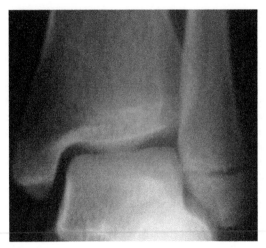

Fig. 1. D-W type A.

displacement, and external rotation on contact pressure in the ankle joint. Their findings suggest that all these factors, especially shortening, increase contact pressures across the midlateral and posterior-lateral talar dome.[38,56] Curtis[56] expanded the study and found that a lateral malleolar fracture can have devastating effects on the ankle, even if the deltoid is intact. For these reasons, the author routinely repairs all complete, even minimally displaced, lateral malleolar fractures surgically, assuming the patient is a surgical candidate.

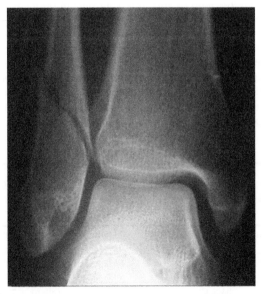

Fig. 2. D-W type B.

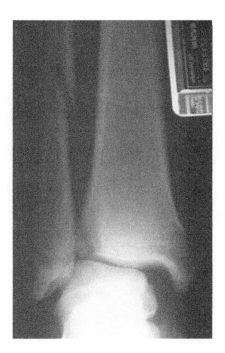

Fig. 3. D-W type C.

DANIS-WEBER TYPE A FRACTURES

D-W type A avulsion fractures of the lateral malleolus are seldom displaced and usually stable. These fractures correspond to Lauge-Hansen supination-adduction (SAD) injuries. The mechanism of injury involves inversion, causing either a rupture of the lateral collateral ligaments or a transverse, avulsion fracture of the lateral malleolus. If the inversion force continues, the talus tilts medially until it contacts and fractures the medial malleolus by shearing it off. This produces a short, vertical medial malleolar fracture, the classic finding of the SAD stage II, which is tricky to fixate precisely (**Fig. 4**).[38]

Some investigators believe that isolated fibular D-W type A fractures are amenable to conservative treatment by short leg non–weight-bearing immobilization.[32] Pakarinen and colleagues[51] found that isolated lateral malleolar fractures in an otherwise stable mortise could be treated successfully without surgical reduction and that post-treatment fibular displacement did not cause functional impairment or pain. If patient noncompliance or signs of delayed or nonunion are noted, surgical correction by single intramedullary screw, placed either by open or percutaneous technique, is warranted and usually successful. The technique is similar to the technique used in Jones fractures of the fifth metatarsal. The screw should ideally purchase the medial cortex of the proximal fibula rather than float in the cancellous bone. Due to the transverse nature of this avulsion fracture, conventional interfragmentary fixation is usually not possible. If necessary, a distal fibular buttress plate may be used. AcuMed also offers a fibular rod which, placed intramedullary, is useful in this situation. Once the fibula is stabilized, ligamentotaxis should help to reduce the medial malleolus, if fractured. The author routinely repairs these medial malleolar fractures with 2 cannulated, cancellous screws, if the size of the medial malleolar fragment allows, inserted perpendicular to the fracture line. These screws do not need to purchase the far

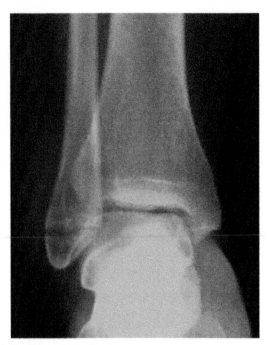

Fig. 4. D-W type A fibular avulsion fracture.

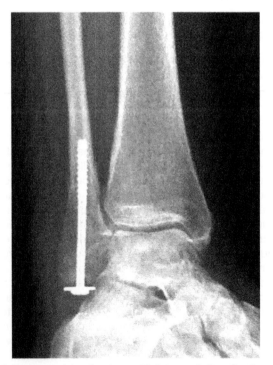

Fig. 5. D-W type A fibular avulsion fracture with intramedullary fixation.

cortex, unless the bone is osteoporotic[57]: 40% to 45% of these fractures have related osteochondral lesions that need to be investigated and possibly repaired.[6] D-W type A/SAD fractures rarely result in trimalleolar fractures (**Fig. 5**).

OVERVIEW OF BIMALLEOLAR AND BIMALLEOLAR EQUIVALENT FRACTURES

With failure of the medial ligaments or fracture of the medial malleolus, the game changes. No longer is conservative therapy sufficient to stabilize and maintain reduction of the ankle mortise; surgical intervention is imperative. Even a simple D-W type A avulsion fracture of the distal fibula becomes difficult to close-reduce in the face of a medial malleolar fracture or deltoid compromise.[57] Isolated fractures of the medial malleolus are rare and often accompany occult fractures of the distal fibula or come in the wake of chronic lateral ankle instability and ligamentous laxity.

Yablon and colleagues,[36] in their research in 1976, established the guidelines that are still in use today that justify surgical intervention in bimalleolar ankle fractures. Yablon and colleagues proposed, "The reason why late degenerative arthritis developed in some patients who had sustained displaced bimalleolar fractures of the ankle was investigated. The roentgenograms indicated that incomplete reduction of the lateral malleolus and a residual talar tilt were present...We concluded that the lateral malleolus is the key to the anatomic reduction of bimalleolar fractures, because the displacement of the talus faithfully followed that of the lateral malleolus." Yablon and colleagues thus elevated the role of the fibula from muscular attachment site to dominant fracture in the ankle fracture complex. Before their research, the medial malleolus was the focus of the effort in reducing ankle fractures and re-establishing anatomic alignment.[58,59] In 2003, Michelson challenged the long-standing gospel of the lateral malleolus. Michelson[60] stated, "Although some early work suggested that the lateral malleolus was the key to ankle stability, recent investigations have conclusively demonstrated that it is not."[60,61] He goes on to propose that the primary stabilizer of the ankle under load is the deltoid complex. Rupture of the deltoid allows abnormal motion of the talus, and stabilization of the fibula does not completely correct this motion. Michelson even asserts, "Completely removing the fibula will not result in any talar displacement with respect to the tibia. Therefore, if the talus is not anatomically located in the mortise, the medial structures must be compromised. Observation of such a displaced talus is de facto evidence of an unstable ankle injury."[60]

Bimalleolar equivalent fractures are those fractures where, instead of medial malleolar fracture, deltoid ligament rupture occurs. Thordarson states, "Less stability is present in patients with deltoid ligament rupture rather than a medial malleolus fracture, because internal fixation of the medial malleolar fragment does restore some degree of medial stability via the attached deltoid ligament." As Yablon and colleagues[36] discovered, "the lateral malleolus is the key to the anatomic reduction of displaced bimalleolar fractures, and that restoring the integrity of the lateral malleolus establishes stability of the ankle." Given that the talus follows the fibula, the talus is restored to its correct position once the fibula is anatomically reduced. This also returns the medial structures to their proper positions, allowing the deltoid to heal without surgical repair. If more than 2 mm of medial clear space remains after fibular reduction, however, then the medial side should be explored for blockage (**Fig. 6**).[62,63]

At Broadlawns Medical Center, the deltoid ligament on displaced, bimalleolar fractures is not routinely repaired. The author does, however, perform open reduction instead of percutaneous repair of medial malleolar fractures. In one case where percutaneous fixation of what seemed a satisfactorily reduced medial malleolar fracture was

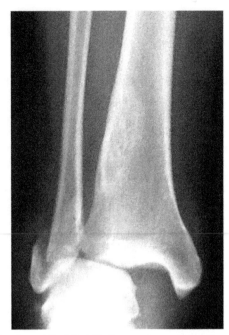

Fig. 6. Distal fibular fracture with deltoid failure: note medial gutter space widening. Bimalleolar equivalent fracture.

attempted, the fracture fragment seemed to become more displaced as the screw was tightened. Finally, opening the medial side revealed that the medial malleolar fracture fragment, although it looked well aligned on C-arm, was rotated 90°, with the cancellous fracture surface facing medially. The author has also experienced the traditional Coonrad-Bugg trap, where interposition of the posterior tibial tendon prevents reduction of the medial malleolar fracture fragment.[64] While open reducing the medial malleolar fracture, if the fibers of a ruptured deltoid ligament hinder the anatomic reduction, they are primarily repaired but repair is not performed routinely. Studies have also supported this thinking, showing no benefit, no increased stability, or no improvement in long-term results, with primary repair of the deltoid.[6]

DANIS-WEBER TYPE B FRACTURES

D-W type B distal fibular fractures are usually spiral oblique or oblique fractures, often showing lateral displacement and/or shortening of the distal fibular fracture fragment. These fractures correspond to the Lauge-Hansen supination-external rotation (SER) and pronation-abduction (PAB) injuries (**Figs. 7** and **8**).

D-W Type B/SER

The mechanism of injury involved in the D-W type B/SER fracture is external rotation. First, the anterior-inferior tibiofibular ligament (AITFL) ruptures or, occasionally, avulses one of its insertions on the tibia (Tillaux-Chaput fracture) or the fibula (Wagstaffe fracture). Further rotation causes the spiral oblique fracture of the fibula seen in response to a twisting force. This fracture usually starts anteriorly where the fibula is overlapped by the anterior lateral tubercle of Chaput of the tibia. Because the fibula is locked in place in the fibular notch of the tibia by the surrounding bony architecture,

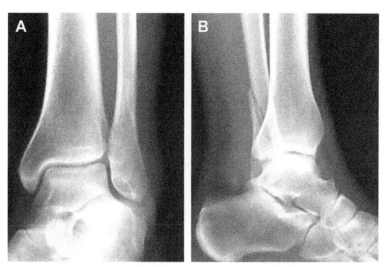

Fig. 7. D-W type B oblique fibular fracture preoperatively. Note misleading anteroposterior view (*A*) compared with lateral view (*B*).

the force of the injury follows the path of least resistance through the fibular bone. Further rotation either ruptures the posterior-inferior tibiofibular ligament (PITFL) or causes avulsion fracture of the posterior lateral tubercle of the tibia (posterior malleolus or Volkmann fracture). Finally, the medial deltoid ligament fails or the medial malleolus is avulsed (**Fig. 9**).

The spiral oblique fracture pattern lends itself well to interfragmentary screw fixation. A long fracture line can even accommodate multiple interfragmentary screws. Using lag screws or lag technique avoids screw threads crossing the fracture and distracting it. There are many anatomic, locking plates currently on the market that provide ease of fixation in these cases. The favorite at Broadlawns Medical Center

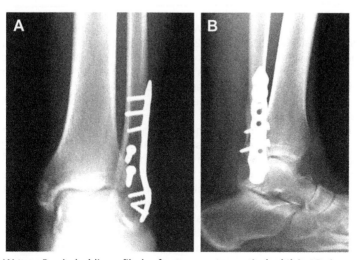

Fig. 8. D-W type B spiral oblique fibular fracture postoperatively. (*A*) is AP view and (*B*) is lateral view.

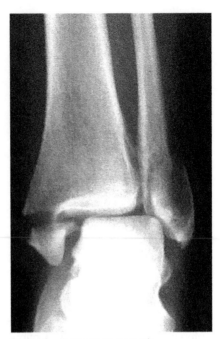

Fig. 9. D-W type B bimalleolar fracture preoperatively.

is the US Implant distal fibular locking plate. This plate includes a dynamic hole in the proximal aspect of the plate for use in applying small amounts of compression or distraction, as needed. The plate allows multiangle locking capability in most holes. The author commonly uses at least 2 locking screws distal to the fracture line and 1 or 2 locking screws proximal to the fracture line (the remainder being nonlocking, cortical screws). Cortical screws, inserted before any locking screws, tighten the plate against the bone; then, locking screws can be inserted. This produces a stable construct. Another useful technique, if the fracture line is proximal enough to the joint, is to insert a cortical screw through both cortices, distal to the fracture line. This screw must avoid invading the lateral gutter. When the author was first introduced to the US Implant distal fibular plate, the screws, 2.7 mm and 3.0 mm, seemed too small, but the author has been using this plate for more than 4 years with not a single incidence of hardware loosening or failing. It helps that this hardware is titanium. It only takes one patient with a legitimate nickel allergy to reconsider using stainless steel. There are also many other titanium, low-profile, locking, distal fibular plates available, which perform equally well (**Fig. 10**).

With failure of the medial structures, the lateral shoulder of the talar dome can contact the tibial plafond, causing potential osteochondral damage. Medial failure leads to a potentially unstable ankle joint and can increase the possibility of dislocation.[38] As discussed previously, the medial malleolar avulsion fracture is reduced and fixated with 1 partially threaded, cancellous, cannulated screw or 2, depending on the size of the medial malleolar fragment. Satisfactory fixation can be accomplished with a single screw. Any compromise to rotational stability from using a single screw is offset by avoiding comminution of a small medial malleolar fragment by overzealous screw placement. Alternatively, the medial malleolus can be fixated in a tension band wiring technique.[57] D-W type B/SER fractures can also produce either failure of the PITFL or avulsion fracture of the posterior-lateral tibial tubercle/posterior malleolus (**Fig. 11**).

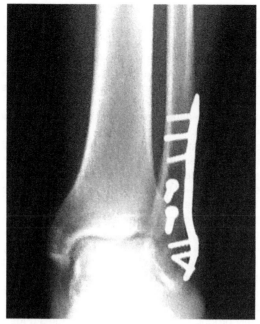

Fig. 10. Double interfragmentary compression screws.

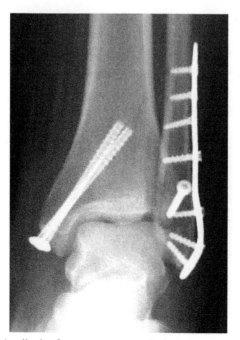

Fig. 11. D-W type B bimalleolar fracture postoperatively.

D-W Type B/PAB

The mechanism of injury involved in the D-W type B/PAB fracture causes medial injury first due to the pronated position of the foot. Either medial deltoid ligament rupture or avulsion fracture of the medial malleolus occurs. Abduction then causes rupture of the AITFL and/or the PITFL or avulsion fractures of their insertions. The resulting instability of the distal fibular fragment allows a short oblique (sometimes transverse) fracture of the fibula. If abductory force continues, the distal fibular fracture fragment has an impact on the proximal fibula, causing the trademark butterfly fragment seen in this fracture type (**Figs. 12** and **13**).

Merrill[65] observed that the interosseous membrane (IOM) is sensitive to abductory forces and may be compromised. As in the SER, the lateral shoulder of the talar dome can crush on contact with the tibial plafond, causing osteochondral lesion. The fibular fractures associated with the D-W type B/PAB injury are more difficult to reduce and fixate due to their nearly transverse nature. The butterfly fragment, if present, further complicates the reduction. Cerclage wire may be needed to hold the butterfly fragment in position, and interfragmentary screw fixation may or may not be possible. Either an anatomic distal fibular plate or a one-third tubular plate may be used to maintain position of the fracture fragments. Occasionally, if reduction of the comminuted fragments is impossible, the fibular fracture must be bridged by a longer plate, with sufficient screw fixation proximal and distal to the fracture to provide rigid fixation.[57] The medial malleolus is reduced and fixated (as described previously). D-W type B/PAB fractures rarely produce posterior malleolar fractures (**Figs. 14** and **15**).

In the author's practice, D-W type B fractures make up more than 75% of the ankle fractures seen, with the fracture line almost invariably commencing from the tubercle of Chaput. With few exceptions, all D-W type B fractures are fixed surgically, as long

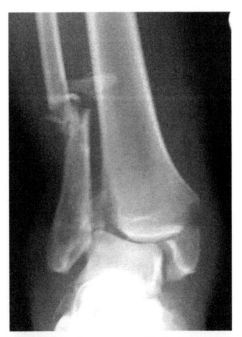

Fig. 12. D-W type C bimalleolar fracture preoperatively. Note the comminuted fibula and horizontal butterfly fragment. Also, anterolateral tibial fracture fragment.

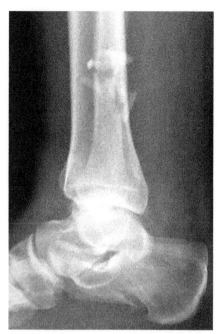

Fig. 13. D-W type C bimalleolar fracture preoperatively. Note the associated calcaneal fracture after fall from the top of a ladder.

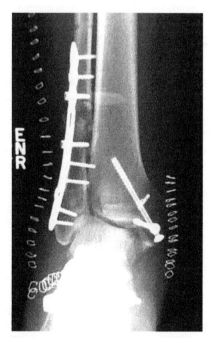

Fig. 14. D-W type C bimalleolar fracture postoperatively. Note proximal screw hole from free screw used to re-establish fibular length and ZipTight trans-syndesmotic fixation. Anteroposterior screw in medial malleolar fragment to fixate longitudinal fracture of malleolus.

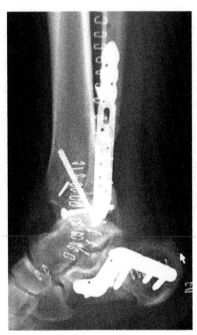

Fig. 15. D-W type C bimalleolar fracture postoperatively. Note Tornier Wave Plate used for calcaneal fixation.

as patients are surgical candidates. Although there is compelling research to support conservative treatment of many D-W type B fractures,[66] the author's unique and often multiply comorbid, noncompliant patient population continues to legitimize the choice of operative treatment.

OVERVIEW OF TRIMALLEOLAR AND TRIMALLEOLAR EQUIVALENT FRACTURES

Rarely (1% of all reported ankle fractures) truly isolated posterior malleolar fractures are experienced, although they are present 7% to 44% of the time in combination with other ankle fractures.[67,68] A high index of clinical suspicion is required to rule out occult fracture of the lateral malleolus or Maisonneuve fracture in the face of apparently isolated posterior malleolar fracture.[37] When they do occur, isolated posterior malleolar fractures are a result of axial loading or anterior dislocation of the tibia over a fixed foot.[57] Likewise, isolated anterior distal tibial lip fractures are also uncommon and due to axial loading or dislocation of the tibia posteriorly over a fixed foot.[57]

A generally accepted guideline for fixation of the posterior malleolus is involvement of 25% of the articular surface or when the fragment is displaced more than 2 mm.[57] Assessing the size of the posterior malleolar fracture fragment is often difficult, because a lateral radiograph may not show its true size due to the oblique fracture orientation. CT scans are helpful in evaluating not only the size of the fragment but also any step-off in the joint articular surface.[69] The author has begun to order CT on all trimalleolar fractures so that an educated decision can be made regarding possible fixation of the fragment. Macko and colleagues[70] noted a 35% loss of ankle contact with posterior malleolar fracture involving 50% of the distal tibial surface. Posterior subluxation of the talus and post-traumatic degenerative joint disease (DJD) was shown in some studies when the posterior malleolar fragment exceeded 25% of the joint surface and was not anatomically reduced.[18,24,71,72] In 1988, Harper and Hardin[73] found that the poor results may have been due to inadequate reduction of medial and lateral fractures associated with the posterior malleolar fracture, which were usually treated nonoperatively. They also found that, if the fibula was anatomically reduced and properly fixated, it returns the talus and the posterior malleolus to their anatomic positions in fractures where the posterior malleolus made up 25% to 45% of the joint surface, with no difference in the results between those posterior malleolar fractures that were fixated and those that were not.[73] Carr[74] found, in 2003, that, "in most ankle fractures involving a posterior fragment, the PITFL can be repaired by reduction and fixation of a posterolateral avulsion fracture of the distal tibia, thus providing fixation of the syndesmosis, and eliminating the need for syndesmosis transfixation.[74] Mingo-Robinet and colleagues[75] concluded from their study of posterior malleolar fractures that, "[open reduction and internal fixation] ORIF of the posterior malleolar fragment of a trimalleolar ankle fracture is warranted if anatomic reduction is not achieved via closed reduction," and that, "these results encourage us to fix all fragments of more than 25% of the articular surface, and to reduce and fix most of the smaller fragments that cannot be satisfactorily reduced by ligamentotaxis" (**Figs. 16** and **17**).

After reduction of the dominant fibular fracture and any medial fracture, posterior malleolar fractures can be approached from posterior to anterior or vice versa. Posterior approach involves dissection between the peroneal tendons and the Achilles tendon. Reduction is maintained temporarily by Kirschner wires (K-wires) and then 1 or 2 cannulated, cancellous screws, inserted perpendicular to the fracture line, complete the fixation.[57] Alternatively, the fragment can be approached from the anterior ankle, fixated via percutaneous screw placement or through the incision used for medial malleolar repair, depending on the orientation of the fracture. Care must be taken in this technique to ensure that the fragment is not displaced posteriorly by

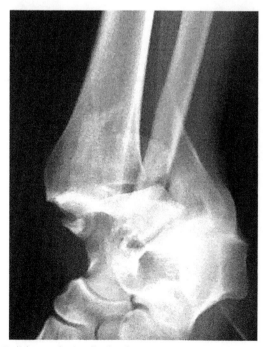

Fig. 16. D-W type B dislocated trimalleolar fracture preoperatively.

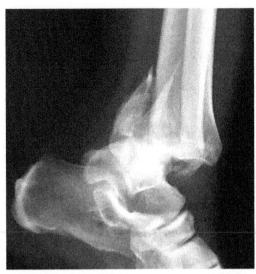

Fig. 17. D-W type B dislocated trimalleolar fracture preoperatively lateral view.

screw insertion and that the fragment is sufficiently large that the screw threads do not cross the fracture, thus distracting it. If necessary, some threads can be cut from the end of a longer-than-measured screw to keep the threads within the posterior malleolar fragment.[76,77] The author usually uses the anterior approach if fixation of the posterior malleolus is necessary (**Figs. 18** and **19**).

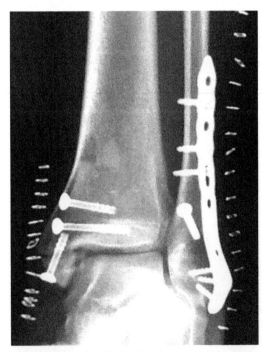

Fig. 18. D-W type B dislocated trimalleolar fracture postoperatively. Note comminuted medial malleolar fragment with both vertical shear and horizontal avulsion components.

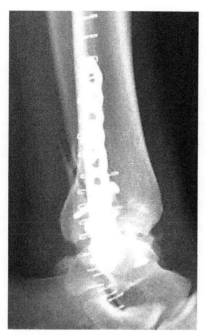

Fig. 19. D-W type B dislocated trimalleolar fracture postoperatively. Note inadequate reduction of posterior fibular spike.

DANIS-WEBER TYPE C FRACTURES

D-W type C/PER fractures also begin medially, with pronation causing either deltoid failure or avulsion of the medial malleolus. Next, the AITFL ruptures or avulses its insertions, allowing external rotation to fracture the fibula in the classic high, spiral, oblique backward fracture pattern, with the fracture line running from posterior-inferior to anterior-superior. Rupture of the PITFL or posterior malleolar fracture ensues. Because this mechanism can also be responsible for high SER-type or Maisonneuve fractures, apparently isolated medial or posterior malleolar fractures (both of which are rare) should make physicians suspicious of high fibular fracture.[37] These fractures are amenable to interfragmentary screw placement and either anatomic or one-third tubular plating. If a fracture is long and unstable and a single plate does not provide sufficient resistance to bending stress, 2 one-third tubular plates can be stacked so that they overlap by several holes. It is often in these types of fractures that significant shortening of the distal fibular fracture fragment may be encountered. A bone clamp on the distal fragment, applying distraction, can be used to restore the fibular length. Restoration can then be temporarily maintained by K-wires or Steinmann pins driven through the distal fibular fragment into the distal tibia or talus. If this is unsuccessful, the chosen plate can be fixed to the distal fibular fragment with 2 screws and a free screw (2 mm longer than measured) inserted bicortically into the proximal fibular fragment, proximal to the plate. A lamina spreader is then used between the free screw and proximal end of the plate to drive the fracture fragment distally, restoring the fibula to length, while the proximal aspect of the plate is temporarily clamped to capture the reduction. D-W type C/PER fractures can also produce failure of the PITFL or avulsion of the posterior malleolus (**Figs. 20–23**).

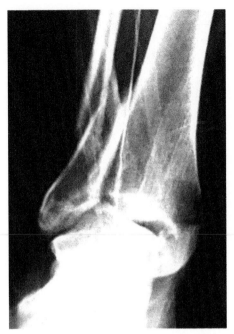

Fig. 20. D-W type C dislocated trimalleolar fracture preoperatively.

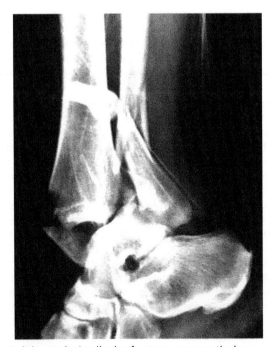

Fig. 21. D-W type C dislocated trimalleolar fracture preoperatively.

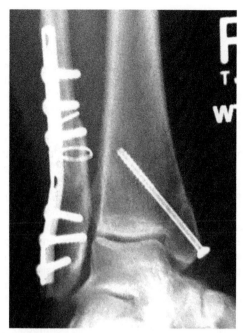

Fig. 22. D-W type C dislocated trimalleolar fracture postoperatively. Note cerclage wire fixation of comminuted fibular fracture.

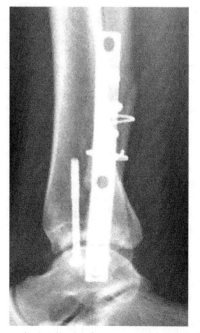

Fig. 23. D-W type C dislocated trimalleolar fracture postoperatively.

PROXIMAL FIBULAR/MAISONNEUVE FRACTURES

Maisonneuve[78] was the first to compare the ankle joint to the carpentry mortise and tenon joint. He was also the first to recognize that the integrity of the syndesmotic ligaments combined with the external rotational forces applied to the ankle dictated the fracture pattern. There has been much controversy surrounding the actual pathomechanics of the Maisonneuve proximal fibular fracture. It may make intuitive sense to picture complete disruption of the syndesmotic complex as the prerequisite to the proximal fibular fracture, but this may not always be the case.

In discussing the Maisonneuve fracture, review the anatomy of the syndesmotic complex. Distally, the inferior tibiofibular joint includes the fibular notch in the tibia, in which the fibula is firmly locked by several ligaments.[79–82] This articulation between the tibia and fibula is reinforced by the AITFL, the interosseous ligament (IOL), the distal IOM, the PITFL superficially, and the transverse tibiofibular ligament (TTFL) deep to it.[79–85] It is author's opinion that the TTFL is more important in maintaining the posterior integrity of the tibiofibular and tibiotalar articulations than often thought. The thick, twisting fibers of the TTFL attach across the entire posterior aspect of the distal tibia, below the posterior tibial margin, helping to prevent posterior dislocation of the talus and effectively deepening the mortise, increasing the stability of the ankle joint.[83,86,87] The IOL is actually a thickening of the distal IOM and acts as a spring, allowing the tibia and fibula to spread apart during dorsiflexion of the ankle to accommodate the talus, which is wider anteriorly.[81,83–87]

Ogilvie-Harris and colleagues[85] studied the relative contribution of each component of the distal syndesmotic complex to resistance to lateral fibular displacement. They found that the AITFL provided 35% resistance to displacement, the TTFL 33%, the IOL 22%, and the PITFL 9%. Injury to one or more of these ligaments results in instability of the joint and abnormal articular relationships and motion.[85]

In 1840, Maisonneuve[78] postulated that external rotation of the foot was a mechanism of injury in ankle fracture. He concluded that if the AITFL were intact, then an oblique fracture of the lateral malleolus would ensue. If the AITFL ruptured, there would be a fracture of the proximal third of the fibula, the fracture that bears his name. In 1976, Pankovich[88] at Cook County Hospital reported on 17 cases of Maisonneuve fracture (which he stated made up 5% of all ankle fractures seen in their emergency department) and reported that most had the classic Maisonneuve fracture pattern of anterior-superior to posterior-inferior and that some had the classic SER pattern of anterior-inferior to posterior-superior. In those fractures that Pankovich repaired surgically, he found rupture of the IOL in every fracture, suggesting that the IOL ruptured in the early stages of these injuries, which is contrary to the findings of Lauge-Hansen. In Pankovich's associated cadaveric experimentation, after sectioning of the AITFL, external rotation produced rupture of the IOL and a Maisonneuve-type fracture of the proximal fibula. When the AITFL and IOL were sectioned first, external rotation produced the SER-type proximal fibular fracture. The IOM remained intact in all attempts. Pankovich hypothesized that IOM rupture was a late-stage finding in this type of fracture, resulting from a lateral displacement force on the IOM.[88]

Bonnin[59] found in 1950 that the IOL, IOM, and PITFL remained intact in all Maisonneuve fractures, which was in opposition to Pankovich's operative findings. Wilson[89] stated in 1984 that, "in general, the more proximal the fibula fracture, the greater the damage to the tibiofibular ligaments. The most extensive tearing is found with…Maisonneuve fractures in which the IOM is usually torn as far proximally as the fibular fracture." Merrill[65] put forth in 1991 that the "posterior hinge," as described by Maisonneuve, in the proximal fibular fracture is, the PITFL and the TTFL. Even when the posterior malleolus fractures, the TTFL remains intact, supporting the posterior syndesmosis, because it inserts across the entire posterior aspect of the tibia. Merrill[65] states that the IOL does little to resist rotational force, so remains intact as the fibula rotates externally: "The proximal fibula fracture occurs when the rotation of the fibula is prevented by the capsuloligamentous structures of the proximal tibiofibular joint." Merrill also noted, "The IOM was easily disrupted by applying an abduction force to the distal fibula."

So, where Pankovich called Maisonneuve fractures "a severe injury to the ankle, which includes complete diastasis," and Geissler and colleagues[57] stated, "Fractures associated with syndesmotic disruption are usually unstable and often require operative stabilization," Merrill concluded that "the Maisonneuve fracture can, and often does occur with a partial syndesmotic diastasis. These injuries are relatively stable, and they can be treated non-operatively by internally rotating the foot and thus using the posterior hinge...yielding an anatomic reduction." According to Court-Brown and colleagues,[6] "The use of MRI scanning has confirmed an inconstant relationship between the location of the fibular fracture and the extent of IOM damage...In D-W Type C fractures, abduction forces cause rupture of the IOM to the level of the fracture, but in pure external rotation injuries, this does not occur and the IOM is mainly intact, especially if the fracture is at the level of the fibular neck. In injuries caused by both external rotation and abduction forces, the extent of IOM damage varies." Court-Brown and colleagues[6] also noted, as commonly observed by lower extremity surgeons, that, "It is interesting to note that suprasyndesmotic fibular fractures do not occur between a point about 12–15 cm above the ankle and the fibular neck."

So, the pendulum of thought on Maisonneuve fractures has swung, and the current thinking is that complete rupture of the entire syndesmotic complex is not necessarily the precursor to proximal fibular fracture. There is recognized consensus that proximal fibular Maisonneuve-type fractures, without medial ankle derangement, do not require surgical intervention. Attempts at ORIF of such fractures could result in damage to the common peroneal nerve. A report in 2011 by Stufkens and colleagues[90] produced treatment recommendations: (1) the medial malleolus should be fixated if fractured; (2) the torn deltoid ligament does not need to be primarily repaired; (3) syndesmotic instability can be treated by placement of one or two tricortical or quadracortical screws, which can be placed percutaneously; and (4) the proximal fibular fracture does not require ORIF. This author recommend non–weight-bearing, long leg casting of extensive or displaced proximal fibular fractures with no other distal sequelae. Occasionally, isolated Maisonneuve fractures that are nondisplaced are treated by neoprene knee sleeve immobilization, to good result. In those rare, high SER fractures of the proximal fibula, where disruption of the syndesmotic complex is clear, trans-syndesmotic fixation is called for. This can be accomplished via tricortical or quadracortical screw placement or by ZipTight (AcuMed) or TightRope (Arthrex) syndesmotic fusion wire devices. The benefit of these devices versus a trans-syndesmotic screw is that the fusion wire can be left in place indefinitely, allowing weight bearing without removal of the device, thus avoiding additional surgery for the patient. This is due to the fiber wire allowing some play in the tibiofibular relationship, mimicking the IOL spring. The author prefers the ZipTight to the TightRope, because it uses titanium rather than stainless steel, and it uses a cinch device instead of requiring that the fiber wire be tied in a large, bulky knot. The use of these suture button devices was investigated by DeGroot and colleagues[91] in 2011. They reviewed the results of 24 patients treated with the TightRope device over 20 months. Their results showed that syndesmotic reduction was maintained in all patients throughout the follow-up period but that reoperation to remove the device was more common than expected: 25% of patients required removal of the device due to local irritation or lack of motion, 16% had subsidence of the device with local osteolysis, and 12% developed heterotopic ossification within the syndesmotic ligament. This author has had similar results with the TightRope device, but none so far with the ZipTight, and hypothesizes that this is due to the lack of the bulky fiber wire knot.

A related injury, a high ankle sprain or diastasis of the tibial and fibula (syndesmotic ligament disruption without fracture), is rare.[92–94] Edwards and DeLee[93] described the "latent diastasis," which is not appreciated without stress radiographs, and the "frank diastasis," which is obvious on normal radiographs. Often, latent diastasis is only evident after several weeks, when a radiograph reveals ossification of the IOM at the area of injury. Although Gustilo and colleagues[95] and other investigators recommend either cast immobilization or non–weight bearing for several weeks, the author recommends surgical syndesmotic repair via ZipTight or TightRope syndesmotic fusion wire device for symptomatic diastasis (**Fig. 24**).

Syndesmotic compromise should be investigated intraoperatively so that it can be repaired. If the fibular fracture is within 3 cm to 4 cm of the joint, sydesmotic fixation may not be necessary, but all D-W type B, and especially type C, fractures have the potential for syndesmotic instability. Syndesmotic disruption does not necessarily cause ankle joint instability. It has been found that coexistent deltoid rupture is what critically destabilizes the ankle.[96] Testing of the integrity of the syndesmosis via Cotton test, placing a bone hook around the fibula, and applying lateral traction to elicit widening of the mortise can be performed.[57] Alternatively, a modified Cotton test can be performed by internally and externally rotating the foot while observing the mortise on the C-arm to look for widening. A positive result in either test supports fixation of the syndesmosis. In the past, syndesmotic screws were used in 40% of D-W type B fractures and in up to 80% of D-W type C fractures.[14,23,77,97] Currently,

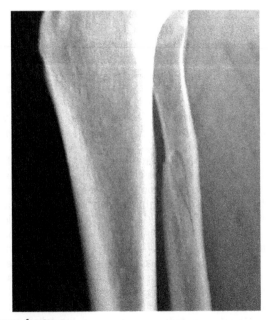

Fig. 24. Maisonneuve fracture.

syndesmotic fixation is called for only when there is persistent syndesmotic disruption, tibiofibular diastasis, or medial ligament failure.[77]

The syndesmosis can be stabilized using a single tricortical or quadracortical screw (multiple screws in diabetic, osteoporotic, or morbidly obese patients) or ZipTight or TightRope syndesmotic fusion wires, placed parallel to the joint surface, with the foot dorsiflexed. It is the author's belief that nonflexible fixation via screws limits the normal motion of the ankle joint and must be removed before a patient resumes weight bearing. Controversy remains over whether trans-syndesmotic screws must be removed.[98] In one study of 52 patients with trans-syndesmotic screws, 52% had intact screws after 1 year, 19% had broken screws, and 29% had undergone elective screw removal.[99] Another recent report showed that retained trans-syndesmotic screws were associated with poor functional outcomes.[100] Studies have also shown that removal of trans-syndesmotic screws allow better ankle range of motion,[101] whereas biomechanical studies of the suture button devices show that they allow "physiologic micromotion" to occur between the tibia and fibula.[102] The syndesmotic fusion wire devices, with their flexibility, do not need to be removed before weight bearing.

Occasionally, the author has seen distal fibular D-W type A and type B fractures with associated Maisonneuve fractures and without complete syndesmotic failure. The author previously postulated that perhaps a separate, blunt trauma caused the proximal fibular fracture. Given that the fibula can externally rotate without compromising the IOM, this could cause the combination fracture. The distal fibular fracture is due to the tubercle of Chaput and associated ligaments locking the distal fibula into the fibular notch of the tibia, and continued external rotation is blocked by the ligamentous structures at the knee, locking the proximal fibula in place, and causing it to fracture. This explains the opposite fracture line orientation in the distal and fibular fractures and the mechanism of these rare, but interesting, fractures (**Fig. 25**).

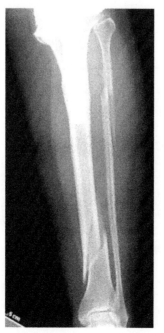

Fig. 25. Combination Maisonneuve proximal and distal fibular fractures.

OPEN ANKLE FRACTURES

Open fractures of the ankle are a surgical emergency. Immediately, they require reduction of dislocations, if necessary, and stabilization/splinting to prevent further damage.[57] Open wounds require tetanus prophylaxis, if appropriate, and antibiotic coverage postoperatively. Geissler and colleagues[57] described 3 stages of treatment of open fractures: débridement, fracture stabilization, and wound closure (**Fig. 26**).

Débridement

Inspection of the wound and removal of any obvious foreign material is followed by flushing the area. The author treats all open fractures to a thorough dowsing with a pulse lavage and, if the environment of the fracture or its gross appearance warrants, uses bacitracin (50–100 mL per 100 mL of saline) in the saline flush. It is said that the solution to pollution is dilution. The pulse lavage not only helps to mechanically débride the wound but also reduces the bacterial load in the wound, helping to minimize the chance of infection. If the wound includes the joint capsule, flush the joint well to avoid leaving loose bodies in the joint space.

Fracture Stabilization

It is suggested that, after the débridement of the wound is complete, the instruments used are removed from the operative field, the surgical team regown and reglove, and the patient be redraped to prevent cross-contamination.[57] Although nothing changes about the reduction and fixation of open fractures versus closed fractures, the approach may need to be adjusted. If possible, the fractures should be approached through the traumatic lacerations, to avoid multiple wounds. It may be necessary to

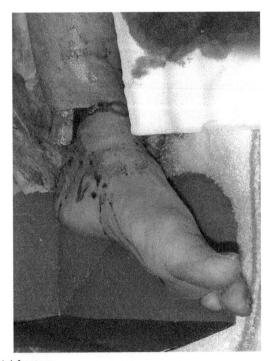

Fig. 26. Open tibial fracture.

extend or connect these lacerations, taking care to avoid islands of skin that may not heal. External fixation and hybrid fixation are also viable options in the complicated open fracture, as is staging of the surgical procedures. Treatment options can include debridement of wounds, application of bridging external fixation, packing the wounds open and revisiting the fracture once the original inflammatory response has subsided.

Wound Closure

It is always preferable to close some soft tissue over any hardware, but if this is not possible, that does not contraindicate internal fixation.[57] If the surgery is performed within the golden period postinjury and cleansing of the wound was thought satisfactory, the author has no problem primarily closing all incisions and lacerations, if possible. Wound Vac/negative-pressure wound therapy in conjunction with skin grafting may also be considered if large soft tissue defects are present.

SURGICAL TIMING

The stages of healing are the inflammatory phase, the proliferative phase, and the reparative phase. It has long been the clinical opinion of the author that, unless there is circulatory impairment, open fracture, unstable dislocation, or the threat of soft tissue necrosis, surgical treatment of ankle fractures should be postponed to allow the soft tissue envelope time to recover from the initial trauma. Soft tissue damage may be less obvious in patients with closed fractures but is no less important. Do not overlook the importance of soft tissue injury in the eventual healing of the fracture.[103] The author's patients are routinely placed in Jones compression dressings and posterior splints, kept non–weight bearing, and placed on the surgical schedule for the next week. In those ankle fractures that have been taken to the operating room emergently, lower extremity surgeons often encounter still-active bleeding and hemorrhagic tissue, engorgement of the soft tissue from the initial inflammatory phase, and difficulty in differentiating tissue planes. There is research evidence to support what has been observed clinically (**Figs. 27** and **28**).

Geissler and colleagues[57] in 1996 stated, "Ankle swelling may peak in 1–7 days, and operative treatment is best done before the period of maximal swelling of after the initial swelling has resolved…No adverse effect has been noted from a delay in surgery, provided that an anatomic reduction is eventually obtained." According to Tull and Borrelli[104] in 2003, "The response of soft tissue to blunt injury involves microvascular and inflammatory processes that produce localized tissue hypoxia and acidosis." Schaser and colleagues[105] stated, "It is shown that initial trauma-induced

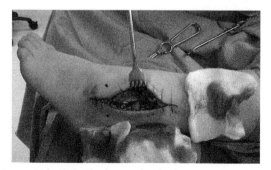

Fig. 27. Early fracture repair. Note the hemorrhagic tissue.

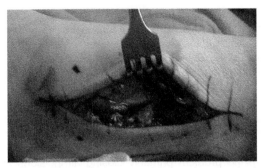

Fig. 28. Early fracture repair. Note obliteration of tissue planes and edema.

microcirculatory disturbances and leukocyte activation lead to a significant impairment in early bone healing...by which soft tissue trauma is linked to decreased fracture healing response in presence of concomitant severe soft tissue damage." In 1961, Tonna and Cronkite[106] reported that the initial cellular reaction to skeletal trauma was generalized to the area surrounding the fracture. They also observed a white cell and fluid infiltrate from the surrounding soft tissue and damaged vessels into the muscle and soft tissue surrounding the fracture, along the whole length of the bone. The peak of this activity occurred at 32 hours after the trauma. Five days after the trauma, the potential for this proliferative behavior was similar to that in any nonfractured bone.[106] The author proposes that it is best to perform surgical treatment of ankle fractures at least 5 days postinjury. Delaying the surgery not only avoids additional tissue damage during the inflammatory phase but also then serves to jump start the stalled proliferative phase of healing, aiding in the ensuing bone healing.

COMPLICATIONS

Post-traumatic DJD or osteoarthritis (OA) is the most common postoperative complaint after ankle fracture.[38] The more severe the fracture, the more likely a patient develops DJD.[107] Beris and colleagues[108] reported that DJD was more common in bimalleolar fractures than in isolated malleolar fractures and that there was no significant difference in the occurrence between bimalleolar and trimalleolar fractures. OA developed in 3.7% of unimalleolar fractures, 20.7% of bimalleolar fractures, and 29% of trimalleolar fractures. The size of the posterior malleolar fracture fragment also determined the likelihood of OA. For posterior malleolar fractures comprising up to 25% of the joint surface, DJD was found in 26.2% of patients; for fragments larger than 25% of the joint surface, DJD was seen in 35% of patients. In general, the incidence of DJD is significantly lower in patients who had good to excellent anatomic reduction of their fractures than in those with fair to poor surgical results.[38]

The incidence of delayed unions and nonunions in ankle fractures is relatively low, ranging from 0.9% to 1.9%.[109] Most often, it is the medial malleolus that fails to show complete union, usually due to soft tissue interposition or inadequate fixation.[110]

Patients with systemic comorbidities also need special consideration. Diabetes, peripheral vascular disease, nicotine dependence, osteoporosis, and obesity are all common issues that may make satisfactory results harder to achieve after ankle fracture repair.[111] A growing population of diabetics in the country will make assessing and accommodating their special needs increasingly more important for trauma surgeons. With the increased risk of infection and hardware failure in diabetics from neuropathy, infection, and poor bone stock comes a greater burden on surgeons to stack the deck in patients' favor. Bevilacqua and Stapleton[112] observe, "It is unrealistic to expect traditional internal fixation techniques alone to maintain compression...adjusting techniques and using supplemental fixation may enhance osseous stability." The less a surgeon disrupts the soft tissue envelope surrounding a diabetic ankle fracture, the better. This is often achieved by use of percutaneous fixation or a combination of percutaneous and open locking plate fixation.[113] As a rule of thumb, take the already established principles of AO fixation, namely, meticulous dissection, anatomic reduction, rigid fixation, and early mobilization, and beef them up for the at-risk populations with diabetes, osteoporosis, and other healing issues. Specifically, make sure that good compression is achieved across the fractures; use longer locking plates; increase the number of trans-syndesmotic screws or ZipTight fusion wires; consider inserting ZipTight through a washer; or better yet, insert the ZipTight through the plate if possible, to help distribute their pull over a larger area, reducing the chance of subsidence or osteolysis. In cases of poor bone quality, noncompliance with or inability to remain non–weight bearing, neuropathy, or any combination of these factors, hybrid fixation may be called for. This can include a combination of internal and external fixation devices and may even involve extreme temporary fixation in the form of a large Steinmann pin driven from the plantar calcaneus, through the talus, and into the tibia to maintain alignment until bony union is achieved.[57]

It is always important to inform patients preoperatively of the possible postoperative course and potential complications, including, but not limited to, continuing pain, nonunion of bone, painful or failed hardware, need for further surgery, and even limb loss. With high-risk diabetic patients, the need for further surgery is more likely than in healthy patients, as is the possibility of the development of Charcot neuroarthropathy, which could lead to limb loss. This is not to say that conservative treatment is without complication. Cast immobilization of even the most stable ankle fractures is never straightforward in diabetics, especially those with neuropathy. There is no feeling worse than removing a cast from an insensate diabetic with a simple D-W type A fracture and finding a fracture and an ulceration to deal with.

SUMMARY

Although ankle fractures are common, they are seldom routine. This complex, weight-bearing joint's repair can be a challenge for even the most seasoned surgeons. Understanding the mechansim of injury, the pathomechanics and anatomy of the area, and the principles of fixation is key to achieving satisfactory results. The author has found, from research and experience, that although the fibular fracture is a key component of the whole ankle fracture picture, the medial components must not be overlooked. Although some isolated, nondisplaced lateral malleolar fractures may respond well to nonoperative treatment, most ankle fractures are candidates for surgical intervention. Attention must be paid to any associated comorbidities and surgical approach and technique adjusted accordingly. Finally, timing of surgical intervention is crucial not only to making the procedure less challenging technically but also to ensuring better outcomes for patients.

REFERENCES

1. McMulloch PG, Holden P, Robson DJ, et al. The value of mobilization and nonsteroidal anti-inflammatory analgesia in the management of inversion injuries of the ankle. Br J Clin Pract 1985;39:69–72.
2. Ruth CJ. The surgical treatment of injuries of the fibular collateral ligaments of the ankle. J Bone Joint Surg Am 1961;43:229–39.

3. Daly PJ, Fitzgerald RH, Melton LJ, et al. Epidemiology of ankle fractures in Rochester, Minnesota. Acta Orthop Scand 1987;58:539–44.

4. Buddecke DE Jr, Mandracchia VJ, Pendarvis JA, et al. Is this just a sprained ankle? Hosp Med 1998;12:46–52.

5. Phillips WA, Schwartz HS, Keller CS, et al. A prospective randomized study of the management of severe ankle fractures. J Bone Joint Surg Am 1985;67:67–78.

6. Court-Brown C, McQueen MM, Tonetta P III. Ankle fractures in trauma 2006;29:366–82.

7. Flynn JM, Rodriquez-del Rio F, Piza PA. Closed ankle fractures in the diabetic patient. Foot Ankle Int 2000;21:311–9.

8. Muller ME, Nazarian S, Koch P, et al. The comprehensive classification of fractures of long bones. Berlin: Springer-Verlag; 1990.

9. Thordarson DB. Foot and ankle trauma in. Foot and Ankle 2004;14:288–97.

10. Pott P. Some few general remarks on fractures and dislocations. London: Hawes, Clark & Collins; 1768.

11. Lane WA. The operative treatment of fractures. London: Medical Publishing Co; 1910.

12. Lane WA. The operative treatment of simple fractures. London: Medical Publishing Co; 1914.

13. Braunstein PW, Wade PA. Treatment of unstable fractures of the ankle. Ann Surg 1956;149:217–26.

14. Burwell HN, Charnley AD. The treatment of displaced fractures at the ankle by rigid internal fixation and early joint movement. J Bone Joint Surg Br 1965;47:634–60.

15. Charnley J. The closed treatment of common fractures. 3rd edition. Edinburgh (United Kingdom): Livingstone; 1961.

16. Kristensen TB. Treatment of malleolar fractures according to Lauge-Hansen's method: preliminary results. Acta Chir Scand 1949;97:363–79.

17. Magnusson R. On the late results in non-operated cases of malleolar fractures. Acta Chir Scand Suppl 1944;90:1–136.

18. McLaughlin HL. Trauma. Philadelphia: W.B. Saunders; 1960.

19. Watson-Jones R. Fractures and joint injuries. Baltimore (MD): Williams & Wilkins; 1955.

20. Denham RA. Internal fixation for unstable ankle fractures. J Bone Joint Surg Br 1964;46:206–11.

21. Jones WC, Neal EG. Surgery of the fracture of the medial malleolus. South Med J 1962;55:1054.

22. Klossner O. Late results of operative and non-operative treatment of severe ankle fractures. Acta Chir Scand Suppl 1962;293:1–93.

23. Lindsjo U. Operative treatment of ankle fractures. Acta Orthop Scand Suppl 1981;52:1–131.

24. McLaughlin HL, Ryder CT Jr. Open reduction and internal fixation for fractures of the tibia and ankle. Surg Clin North Am 1949;29:1523–34.

25. Svend-Hansen H, Bremerskov V, Baekgaard N. Ankle fractures treated by fixation of the medial malleolus alone. Acta Orthop Scand 1978;49:211–4.

26. Vasli S. Operative treatment of ankle fractures. Acta Chir Scand Suppl 1957;226: 1–74.

27. Danis R, ed. Theorie et pratique de l' osteosynthese. Paris, France: Masson & Cie; 1949.

28. Allgower M, Muller ME, Willenegger H. Technique of internal fixation of fractures. Berlin: Springer-Verlag; 1965.

29. Muller ME, Allgower M, Schneider R, et al. Manual of internal fixation: techniques recommended by the AO-Group. 2nd edition. New York: Springer-Verlag; 1979.
30. Brodie IA, Denham RA. The treatment of unstable ankle fractures. J Bone Joint Surg Am 1974;56:256–62.
31. Cedell CA. Supination-outward rotation injuries of the ankle: a clinical and roentgenological study with special reference to the operative treatment. Acta Orthop Scand Suppl 1967;110:3–148.
32. Hughes JL, Weber H, Willenegger H. Evaluation of ankle fractures. Clin Orthop 1979;138:111–9.
33. Leeds HC, Ehrlich MG. Instability of the distal tibio-fibular syndesmosis after bimalleolar and trimalleolar ankle fractures. J Bone Joint Surg Am 1984;66: 490–503.
34. Ramsey PL, Hamilton W. Changes in tibiotalar area of contact caused by lateral talar shift. J Bone Joint Surg Am 1976;58:356–7.
35. Segal D, Pick RY, Klein HA. The role of the lateral malleolus as a stabilizing factor of the ankle joint: preliminary report. Foot Ankle 1981;2:25–9.
36. Yablon IG, Heller FG, Shouse L. The key role of the lateral malleolus in displaced fractures of the ankle. J Bone Joint Surg Am 1977;57:169–73.
37. Carr JB, Trafton PG. Malleolar fractures and soft-tissue injuries of the ankle. In: Browner BD, Jupiter JB, Levine AM, et al, editors. Skeletal trauma: fractures, dislocations, ligamentous injuries. 2nd edition. Philadelphia: WB Saunders; 1998. p. 2327–97.
38. Mandi DM, Nickles WA, Mandracchia VJ, et al. Ankle fractures. Clin Podiatr Med Surg 2006;23:375–422.
39. Inman VJ. The joints of the ankle. Baltimore (MD): Williams & Wilkins; 1976.
40. Mann RA. Biomechanics of the foot and ankle. In: Mann RA, editor. Surgery of the foot and ankle. 5th edition. St Louis (MO): CV Mosby; 1986. p. 3–43.
41. Bohler L. Diagnosis, pathology and treatment of the os calcis. J Bone Joint Surg Am 1931;13:75.
42. Yablon IG, Segal D, Leach RE. Ankle injuries. New York: Churchill Livingstone; 1983.
43. Joy G, Patzakis MJ, Harvey JP Jr. Precise evaluation of the reduction of severe ankle fractures. Technique and correlation with end results. J Bone Joint Surg Am 1974;56:979–93.
44. Wilson FC, Skilbred LA. Long-term results in the treatment of displaced bimalleolar fractures. J Bone Joint Surg Am 1966;48:1065–78.
45. Zindrick MR, Knight GS, Gogan WJ. The effect of fibular shortening and rotation on the biomechanics of the talocrural joint during various stages of stance phase. Trans Orthop Res Soc 1983;9–136.
46. Cedell CA. Is closed treatment of ankle fractures advisable? [editorial]. Acta Orthop Scand 1985;56:101–2.
47. Chapman MW. Fractures and fracture dislocations of the ankle. In: Mann RA, editor. Surgery of the foot. 5th edition. St Louis (MO): CV Mosby; 1986. p. 568–91.
48. Mast JW, Teipner WA. A reproducible approach to internal fixation of adult ankle fractures; rationale, technique and early results. Orthop Clin North Am 1989;11: 661–79.
49. Pettrone FA, Gail M, Pee D, et al. Quantitative criteria for prediction of the results after displaced fracture of the ankle. J Bone Joint Surg Am 1983;65:667–77.
50. Henderson MS. Trimalleolar fracture of the ankle. Surg Clin North Am 1932;12: 867–72.

51. Pakarinen HJ, Flinkkila TE, Ohtonen PP, et al. Stability criteria for nonoperative ankle fracture management. Foot Ankle Int 2011;32(2):141–7.
52. Weber BG. Die verletzungen des oberen sprunggellenkes: Aktuelle probleme in der chirurgie. Bern (Switzerland): Verlag Hans Huber; 1966.
53. Weber BG. Die verletzungen des oberen sprunggellenkes: Aktuelle probleme in der chirurgie. 2nd edition. Bern (Switzerland): Verlag Hans Huber; 1972.
54. Court-Brown CM, McBirnie J, Wilson G. Adult ankle fractures: an increasing problem? Acta Orthop Scand 1998;69:43–7.
55. Thordarson DB, Motamed S, Hedmand T, et al. The effect of fibular malreduction on contact pressures in an ankle fracture malunion model. J Bone Joint Surg Am 1997;79:1809–15.
56. Curtis MJ, Michelson JD, Urquhart RP, et al. Tibiotalar contact and fibular malunion in ankle fractures. Acta Orthop Scand 1992;63:326–9.
57. Geissler WB, Tsao AK, Hughes JL. Fractures of the ankle. In: Rockwood CA, Green DP, Bucholz RW, et al, editors. Fractures in adults. 4th edition. Philadelphia: Lippincott-Raven; 1996. p. 2202–66.
58. Ashhurst AP, Bromer RS. Classification and mechanism of fractures of leg bones involving the ankle. Arch Surg 1922;4:51–129.
59. Bonnin JG. Injuries to the ankle. London: Heineman; 1950.
60. Michelson JD. Ankle fractures resulting from rotational injuries. J Am Acad Orthop Surg 2003;11:403–12.
61. Michelson JD, Ahn UM, Helgemo SL. Motion of the ankle in a simulated supination-external rotation fracture model. J Bone Joint Surg Am 1996;78:1024–31.
62. Coonrad RW, Bugg EL Jr. Trapping of the posterior tibial tendon and interposition of soft tissue in severe fractures about the ankle joint. J Bone Joint Surg Am 1954;36:744–50.
63. Walker RH, Farris C. Irreducible fracture-dislocations of the ankle associated with interposition of the tibialis posterior tendon. Clin Orthop 1981;160:212–6.
64. Kelikian H, Kelikian AS. Eponymic argot. In: Kelikian H, Kelikian AS, editors. Disorders of the ankle. Philadelphia: WB Saunders; 1985. p. 107–27.
65. Merrill KD. The Maisonneuve fracture of the fibula. Kansas City, MO: Dept of Orthop Surg, Univ of Kansas City; 1991. p. 218–23.
66. Michelson JD, Magid D, Ney DR, et al. Examination of the pathologic anatomy of ankle fractures. J Trauma 1992;32:65–70.
67. DeVries JS, Wijgman AJ, Siervelt IN. Long-term results of ankle fractures with a posterior malleolar fragment. J Foot Ankle Surg 2000;44:211–7.
68. Gale BD, Nugent JF. Isolated posterior malleolar ankle fractures. J Foot Surg 1990;29:80–3.
69. Ferries JS, DeCoster TA, Firoozbakhsh KK, et al. Plain radiographic interpretation in trimalleolar ankle fractures poorly assesses posterior fragment size. J Orthop Trauma 1994;8:328–31.
70. Macko VM, Matthews LS, Swekoski P, et al. The joint contact area of the ankle: the contribution of the posterior malleolus. J Bone Joint Surg Am 1991;73:347–51.
71. McDaniel WJ, Wilson FC. Trimalleolar fractures of the ankle: an end result study. Clin Orthop 1977;122:37–45.
72. Nelson MC, Jensen NK. The treatment of trimalleolar fractures of the ankle. Surg Gynecol Obstet 1942;71:509–14.
73. Harper MC, Hardin G. Posterior malleolar fractures of the ankle associated with external rotation-abduction injuries. J Bone Joint Surg Am 1988;70:1348–56.

74. Carr JB. Malleolar fractures and softl tissue injuries of the ankle. In: Browner BD, Jupiter JB, Levine AM, et al, editors. Skeletal trauma: basic science, management and reconstruction. 3rd edition. Philadelphia: Elsevier Science; 2003. p. 2307–74.

75. Mingo-Robinet J, Lopez-Duran L, Galeote JE, et al. Ankle fractures with posterior malleolar fragment: management and results. J Foot Ankle Surg 2011;50: 141–5.

76. Heim U, Pfeiffer KM. Internal fixation of small fractures: technique recommended by the AO-ASIF Group. 3rd edition. New York: Springer-Verlag; 1988.

77. Mast JW, Teipner WA. A reproducible approach to the internal fixation of adult ankle fractures; rationale, technique and early results. Orthop Clin North Am 1980;11:661–79.

78. Maisonneuve JG. Recherches sur la fracture du perone. Arch Gen Med 1840;7: 165–87 [in French].

79. Vogl TJ, Hochmuth K, Dibold T, et al. Megnetic resonance imaging in the diagnosis of acute injured distal tibiofibular syndesmosis. Invest Radiol 1997;32: 401–9.

80. Ebraheim NA, Lu J, Yang H, et al. Radiographic and CT evaluation of tibiofibular syndesmotic daistasis: a cadaver study. Foot Ankle Int 1997;18:693–8.

81. Grath GR. Widening of the ankle mortise: a clinical and experimental study. Acta Chir Scand Suppl 1995;263(66):1–46.

82. Stiehl JB. Complex ankle fracture dislocations with syndesmotic diastasis. Orthop Rev 1990;19:499–507.

83. Sarrafian SK. Anatomy of the foot and ankle: descriptive, topographic, functional. 2nd edition. Philadelphia: Lippincott; 1993. p. 159–87, 474–551.

84. Duchesneau S, Fallat LM. The Maisonneuve fracture. J Foot Ankle Surg 1995;34: 422–8.

85. Ogilvie-Harris DJ, Reed SC, Hedman TP. Disruption of the ankle syndesmosis: biomechanical study of the ligamentous restraints. Arthroscopy 1994;10: 558–60.

86. Taylor DC, Englehardt DL, Bassett FH III. Syndesmosis sprains of the ankle: the influence of heterotopic ossification. Am J Sports Med 1992;20:146–50.

87. Taylor DC, Bassett FH. Syndesmosis ankle sprains: diagnosing the injury and aiding recovery. Phys Sportsmed 1993;21(12):39–46.

88. Pankovich AM. Maisonneuve fracture of the fibula. J Bone Joint Surg Am 1976; 58:337–42.

89. Wilson FC. Fractures and dislocations of the ankle. In: Rockwood CA, Green DP, editors. Fractures in adults, vol. 2, 2nd edition. Philadelphia: JB Lippincott; 1984. p. 1674.

90. Stufkens SA, van den Bekerom MP, Doornberg JN. Evidence-based treatment of Maisonneuve fractures. J Foot Ankle Surg 2011;50:62–7.

91. DeGroot H, Al-Omari AA, El Ghazaly A. Outcomes of suture button repair of the distal tibiofibular syndesmosis. Foot Ankle Int 2011;32:250–6.

92. Burns BH. Diastasis of the inferior tibiofibular joint. Proc R Soc Med 1943;36: 330.

93. Edwards GS Jr, DeLee JC. Ankle diastasis without fracture. Foot Ankle 1984;4: 305–12.

94. Marymount JV, Lynch MA, Henning CE. Acute ligamentous diastasis of the ankle without fracture. Am J Sports Med 1986;14:407–9.

95. Gustilo RB, Kule RF, Templeman DC. Fractures and dislocations, vol. 2. St Louis (MO): CV Mosby; 1992.

96. Zalavras C, Thordarson D. Ankle syndesmotic injury. J Am Acad Orthop Surg 2007;15:330–9.
97. Grath G. Widening of the ankle mortise: a clinical and experimental study. Acta Chir Scand Suppl 1960;263:1–88.
98. Jones MH, Amendola A. Syndesmosis sprains of the ankle: a systematic review. Clin Orthop Relat Res 2007;455:173–5.
99. Willmott HJ, Singh B, David LA. Outcome and compkications of treatment of ankle diastasis with tightrope fixation. Injury 2009;40(11):1204–6.
100. Moore JA Jr, Shank JR, Morgan SJ, et al. Syndesmosis fixation: a comparison of three and four cortices of screw fixation without hardware removal. Foot Ankle Int 2006;27(8):567–72.
101. Klitzman R, Zhao H, Zhang LQ, et al. Suture-button versus screw fixation of the syndesmosis: a biomechanical analysis. Foot Ankle Int 2010;31(1):69–75.
102. Manjoo A, Sanders DW, Tieszer C, et al. Functional and radiographic results of patients with syndesmotic screw fixation implications for screw removal. J Orthop Trauma 2010;24(1):2–6.
103. Sudkamp NP. Soft-tissue injury: pathophysiology and its influence on fracture management. Evaluation/classification of closed and open injuries. In: AO principles of fracture management. Colton CL, Fernandez Dell'Oca A, Holz U, et al, editors. Stuttgart (Germany), New York: Thieme; 2001;1.5. p. 59–76.
104. Tull F, Borrelli J Jr. Soft-tissue injury associated with closed fractures: evaluation and management. J Am Acad Orthop Surg 2003;11:431–8.
105. Schaser KD, Zhang L, Mittlmeier T, et al. Effect of soft tissue damage on fracture healing: intravital microscopic and biomechanical investigations in rats. Orthop Res Soc 1999;17:678–85.
106. Tonna EA, Cronkite EP. Cellular response to fracture studied with tritiated thymidine. J Bone Joint Surg Am 1961;43:352–62.
107. Broos PL, Bisschop AP. Operative treatment of ankle fractures in adults: correlation between types of fracture and final results. Injury 1991;22:403–6.
108. Beris AE, Kabbani KT, Xenakis TA, et al. Surgical treatment of malleolar fractures: a review of 144 patients. Clin Orthop Relat Res 1997;341:90–8.
109. Lindsjo U. Operative treatment of ankle fracture-dislocations: a follow-up study of 306/321 consecutive cases. Clin Orthop 1985;199:28–38.
110. Mendelsohn MA. Non-union of malleolar fractures of the ankle. Clin Orthop 1965;42:103–18.
111. Haverstock BD, Mandracchia VJ. Cigarette smoking and bone healing: implications in foot and ankle surgery. J Foot Ankle Surg 1998;37:69–73.
112. Bevilacqua NJ, Stapleton JJ. Advanced foot and ankle fixation techniques in patients with diabetes. Clin Podiatr Med Surg 2011;28:661–71.
113. Lee T, Blitz NM, Rush SM. Percutaneous contoured locking plate fixation of the pilon fracture: surgical technique. J Foot Ankle Surg 2008;47:598–602.

Fractures of the Talus: A Comprehensive Review

N. Jake Summers, BS[a], Mica M. Murdoch, DPM[b],*

KEYWORDS

• Talus • Fracture • Ankle • Tarsus

The talus, a critical structure in the ankle and foot, supports normal ambulation and gait in humans. Injury to the talus significantly affects the motion of the foot and ankle, so diagnosing and treating injuries to the talus is crucial. According to Haliburton and Sullivan,[1] the word talus comes from the French *talo*, originating in ancient Greece and Rome. The heel bones of the horse, called *taxillus*, were thrown as dice by the Romans, whereas the Greeks used the vertebrae of sheep, called *astragalus*. The 2 terms were used interchangeably and became associated with the foot bone talus. Talar fractures were identified as early as the sixth century BC. One of the earliest treatments for talar fractures was by Fabricius in 1608, who advocated talectomy. Still practiced today, this procedure is reserved for severe cases.[2] Anderson[3] first coined the term aviator's astragalus, referring to fractures of the talus in World War I pilots in crash landings, when the rudder pedal caused forced dorsiflexion of the foot on impact. The term is still used today.

Talar fractures account for less than 1% of all fractures in the body and between 3% and 6% of fractures in the foot.[4] These fractures are usually high-energy injuries (ie, caused by aviation and automobile accidents). Because of its unique anatomic and functional nature, its multiple articulations, large chondral surface area, and tenuous blood supply, injuries to the talus often cause complications and long-term disability.[5,6] Avascular necrosis and arthritis are common in talar fractures because of neurovascular disruption. Talar fractures are commonly described and classified by their location: head, neck, or body. Depending on the location and type of fracture, treatment and prognosis vary greatly.

ANATOMY OVERVIEW

The talus, a critical link between the leg and the foot, allows the motion needed for ambulation; it is the universal joint of the foot.[1] Serving to support the load of much

a College of Podiatric Medicine and Surgery, Des Moines University, 3200 Grand Avenue, Des Moines, IA 50312, USA
b Broadlawns Medical Center, Des Moines, IA 50314, USA
* Corresponding author.
E-mail address: mmurdoch@broadlawns.org

Clin Podiatr Med Surg 29 (2012) 187–203
doi:10.1016/j.cpm.2012.01.005
0891-8422/12/$ – see front matter Published by Elsevier Inc.

of the body during midstance, it acts as a torque converter for the rotation of the leg to be translated into supinatory and pronatory motion at the subtalar joint.[7]

The talus is the second largest tarsal bone; approximately two-thirds of its surface is covered with articular cartilage. It is stabilized by a combination of joint capsules and ligaments, devoid of muscular attachments. The head of the talus articulates anteriorly with the navicular, and is supported inferiorly by the calcaneonavicular (spring) ligament. The inferior surface of the talus articulates at 3 facets (anterior, middle, and posterior) with the superior surface of the calcaneus. Between the anterior and superior surface lies the tarsal canal, opening laterally to form the tarsal sinus, one of the major routes for blood supply to the talus. The talar dome articulates superiorly with the ankle mortise, including both the medial and lateral malleoli. This surface area is the largest of the articular cartilage and has the greatest range of motion in the foot.

To date, Mulfinger and Trueta[5] have completed the most thorough and complete anatomic study on blood supply to the talus. Because of the high incidence of avascular necrosis in talar fractures, their study was important in determining the extent of vascular disruption to the talus (ie, the risk of avascular necrosis for each type of talar fracture, dislocation, and related soft tissue injuries). Mulfinger and Trueta[5] determined that the main supply of blood to the talus flows through the artery of the tarsal canal from the perforating peroneal and lateral tarsal arteries. This main artery supplies branches to the inferior talar neck, medial talus, and most of the talar body. The remaining portions of the talar head and neck receive their blood supply via the dorsalis pedis artery. The posterior tibial artery is the third major source of blood to the talus and completes the talar blood supply by providing vascularization via its calcaneal branches (**Fig. 1**). Evaluating talar injuries and assessing whether 1 or all of these major sources of blood supply has been compromised helps determine the potential risk of osteonecrosis. With many anastomotic connections between the vessels of the talus, undamaged vessels can aid in providing adequate circulation to the talus after injury.[8]

GENERAL TALAR FRACTURE EVALUATION

In evaluating talar injuries, a thorough medical history should be obtained. Along with this history, it is vital to determine the extent and type of injury and a detailed description of the mechanism of injury. Descriptions of high-energy impacts, such as falls

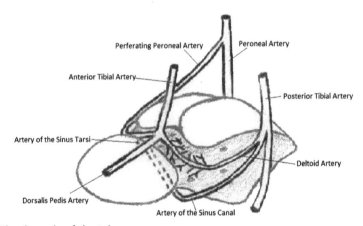

Fig. 1. Blood supply of the talus.

from heights, jumping, landing, and twisting, help determine the degree of injury to the talus. Physical examination findings determine the degree of ecchymosis, swelling, stiffness, and decreased or painful range of motion.

Following initial examinations, standard radiographs identify the specific type of injury. Because of the usual high impacts that cause talar fractures, suspicion for associated spinal injuries should be followed with radiographs.[7] Standard radiographic evaluation of talar fractures should include anteroposterior (AP), oblique, and lateral foot images, as well as an ankle series (AP, mortise, and lateral). The Canale view is often used to evaluate talar head and neck fractures, obtained by placing the beam 15° medially and 75° from the floor. Buckley and Sands[9] also suggest that a computed tomography (CT) scan with accompanying three-dimensional reconstructions should be obtained as a routine part of evaluating talar neck fractures.

TALAR HEAD FRACTURES

Talar head fractures are among the least common fractures of the talus, making up only 10% of all talar fractures.[4,10,11] These fractures are usually a result of either crush or shear injuries. When the talar head becomes locked in the navicular, an axially directed force through the navicular can cause a shearing of the talar head. Compression downward against the sustentaculum tali can break through the articular surface of the talar head, causing comminuted fractures. Coltart[2] described the most likely mechanism of injury to the talar head as a violent, forceful, dorsiflexory force on a fully plantarflexed foot. Because of the lack of muscular attachments to the talus, avulsion type fractures are particularly rare.[2,7] Diagnosis of talar head fracture is based primarily on standard radiographs, including Canale views and possible use of CT imaging in cases in which rotational displacement is suspected.[12,13]

Treatment

Treatment of talar head fracture depends on the degree of comminution, displacement, and stability of the fracture. A regimen of 4 to 8 weeks in a non–weight-bearing, short leg cast with gradual transition to partial and full weight bearing is recommended.[7,14] In the case of unstable fractures, open reduction and internal fixation with K-wires or mini–fragment screws may be necessary. Because of the articulation of the talar head with the navicular, accurate anatomic reduction, achieved through an open or closed technique, is necessary to restore the congruity of the talonavicular joint and reduce the incidence of long-term posttraumatic arthritis and avascular necrosis of the talus. Although avascular necrosis is most commonly associated with fractures of the talar neck, nearly 10% of talar head fractures develop necrosis.[14,15] Surgical intervention of talar head fractures typically consists of fixation via K-wires, subchondral cancellous screws, or bioabsorbable pins, including possible use of bone graft in cases of more severe comminution.[14] Following surgical intervention, patients should be non–weight bearing for a period of 10 to 12 weeks.[12]

TALAR NECK FRACTURES

Approximately 50% of all talar fractures are located within the talar neck. The talar neck is particularly vulnerable to fracture because of its smaller cross-sectional area and thin, weak, cortical bone.[16,17] The most common mechanism of talar fracture is widely accepted as being forced dorsiflexion, described as aviator astragalus by Anderson[3] in 1919 and again by Coltart[2] in 1952. Modern talar neck fractures are usually caused by automobile accidents.[15] This type of fracture is usually preceded by rupture of the posterior subtalar joint ligaments, resulting in impact of the talar neck on the anterior tibia.[3,15,18–20] In severe cases, continued dorsiflexion often causes subluxation of the subtalar joint and, if continued, eventual subluxation of the ankle joint as well. Some evidence suggests a different mechanism of injury, described as a shearing injury caused by application of a plantar axial load while the foot is locked in a plantarflexed position.[21,22]

Talar neck fractures are classified by the displacement of the fracture, combined with any accompanying joint subluxations. The most widely accepted classification system for talar neck fractures was described by Hawkins[23] in 1970 and subsequently modified by Canale[24] in 1990. This classification system describes and defines the injury, and the associated risk of avascular necrosis in each type of talar neck fracture can be estimated. Type I is a nondisplaced fracture without subluxation (**Fig. 2**). Type II is a displaced vertical talar neck fracture with subluxation of the subtalar joint (STJ) (**Fig. 3**). Type III is a displaced vertical talar neck fracture with subluxation of the STJ and tibiotalar (ankle) joint (**Fig. 4**). Type IV is a displaced vertical talar neck fracture with subluxation of the STJ, ankle, and talonavicular joints (**Box 1**).

Although the Hawkins classification seems to be fairly straightforward, there is some discrepancy in the interpretation of the system. For example, it is possible to have a displaced talar neck fracture without the accompanying subluxation of the STJ. Disagreement as to the definition of displaced versus nondisplaced has also led to discussion on how to distinguish between type I and type II fractures.[7] Despite disagreements, the Hawkins classification system remains the universally accepted method to describe talar neck fractures and correlate the injuries with their eventual outcomes.

A significant correlation between the Hawkins classification of a talar neck fracture and the accompanying incidence of avascular necrosis has been reported.[10] The incidence of avascular necrosis associated with talar neck fractures ranges from 0% to 13% for type I, 20% to 50% for type II, 75% to 100% for type III, and approaching 100% for type IV fractures (see **Box 1**).[14] Type I talar neck fractures have a lower risk of avascular necrosis because of the infrequent disruption of blood supply to the talus, with all 3 major sources remaining intact in most cases. Type II fractures can have avascular necrosis in as many as half of all cases, caused by the theoretic disruption of the blood supply through the artery of the tarsal canal and disruption of the interosseous talocalcaneal ligament. Type III neck fractures have a theoretic disruption to the blood supply through both the tarsal canal and the deltoid/calcaneal

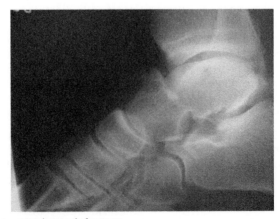

Fig. 2. Hawkins type I talar neck fracture.

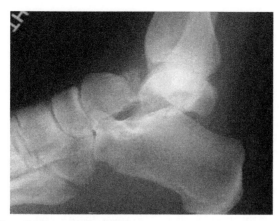

Fig. 3. Hawkins type II talar neck fracture.

branches, thus eliminating both major sources of blood to the body of the talus. In theory, type IV fractures have a disruption of all 3 major sources of blood supply to both the talar body and the head and neck, thus increasing the associated risk of avascular necrosis.

Treatment

Nondisplaced talar neck fractures (type I) are usually treated without surgery, because of the ideal alignment of the joints. Nondisplaced fractures are usually treated for 6 to 8 weeks in a non–weight-bearing, below-knee cast. It is important to continue evaluation of the fracture during treatment with serial radiographs to ensure stability and nondisplacement of the fracture.[14] Patients are typically advanced to partial weight-bearing status, as tolerated, after the initial non–weight-bearing period. Some

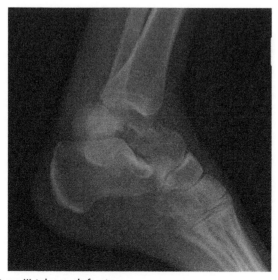

Fig. 4. Hawkins type III talar neck fracture.

> **Box 1**
> **Hawkins classification of talar neck fractures**
>
> Type I: nondisplaced fracture without subluxation; risk of avascular necrosis 0% to 13%
>
> Type II: displaced vertical talar neck fracture with STJ; risk of avascular necrosis 20% to 50%
>
> Type III: displaced vertical talar neck fracture with subluxation of the STJ and tibiotalar (ankle) joint; risk of avascular necrosis 75% to 100%
>
> Type IV: displaced vertical talar neck fracture with subluxation of the STJ, ankle, and talonavicular joint; risk of avascular necrosis 100%

investigators have suggested that internal or external fixation may be necessary to prevent avascular necrosis, but there seems to be no correlation between the rate of talar necrosis and the use of fixation.[16] However, there is some argument that fixation permits earlier range of motion, which has been shown to increase healing of the articular cartilage.[25]

Displaced fractures of the talar neck (types II, III, IV) require operative treatment consisting of initial reduction followed by careful consideration of further intervention. Some investigators have recommended that a closed reduction of the fracture may be all that is necessary to achieve accurate anatomic reduction as well as to relieve any tension on skin and neurovascular impingement to the area.[16] The current recommendation for treating type II, III, and IV talar neck fractures is open reduction and internal fixation (**Fig. 5**).[14] Fractures with rotational or dorsal displacement greater than 5 mm should be treated via open reduction and internal fixation.[4] This provides stability to the area and may aid in preventing articular damage and resultant arthritis to the joints surrounding the talus.

The timing of reduction of talar neck fractures is under debate; some researchers advocate immediate reduction and others argue that reduction is not necessary for at least 24 hours.[16,26] The only consensus seems to be that displaced fractures with resultant skin ischemia that are not amenable to closed reduction are considered

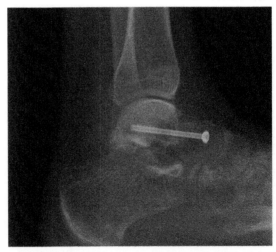

Fig. 5. A talar neck fracture treated by open reduction with internal fixation.

surgical emergencies.[14,27] Thordarson[28] shows that immediate reduction of displaced fractures can prevent severe cases of skin necrosis, particularly in type II and IV fractures, in which the talus can be displaced posteriorly out of the subtalar and ankle joints, compromising the soft tissues and neurovasculature in the area.[14,28]

Open fractures should be treated as emergent. Up to 50% of type II talar neck fractures are open, thus increasing the risk of infection. These types of injuries can have the additional complication of severe postoperative infections, with rates as high as 38%, and a dramatic increase in the rate of surgical failure, leading to complete excision of large fragments of the talus. These cases may require more aggressive, long-term surgical intervention, including fusion, joint replacement, or staged reconstructions.[7,29]

Postoperative management should include a period of non–weight bearing and immobilization, with proper wound care, early range of motion, physical therapy, and eventual progression to weight bearing once radiographic evidence of healing is observed.[8,10]

With the increased incidence of complications after talar neck fractures, treatment can become complex. Injuries with soft tissue damage tend to have an increased rate of these complications.[29] Inherent in soft tissue damage is the potential for osteonecrosis caused by disruption of the blood supply.

After initial treatment, continued radiographic evaluation is necessary to assess stability and continued reduction of the fracture and to monitor signs of osteonecrosis. Bones with intact blood supply typically show evidence of disuse osteoporosis and decreased bone density to the injured area. In the talus, this is most easily recognized in the talar dome as an area of increased radiolucency. This local change in bone density is a positive indication that there is an intact blood supply, and may signify a lower potential for the development of osteonecrosis. This focused radiolucency is known as Hawkins sign, and is a good indicator of intact vasculature.[23,30] The development of Hawkins sign can take from 6 weeks to 3 months.[22] Canale and Beldin[31] showed that the absence of Hawkins sign is not necessarily a highly sensitive method of diagnosing osteonecrosis. Other imaging modalities, including magnetic resonance imaging (MRI) and technetium bone scans, are helpful in determining the presence/absence of viable blood supply and resultant healthy or necrotic bone. Treatment of avascular necrosis can vary widely, from periods of prolonged immobilization and non–weight bearing to ankle and subtalar arthrodesis, depending on the severity of the condition.

TALAR BODY FRACTURES

The body of the talus is responsible for supporting the large axial load during weight bearing and ambulation, with the talar dome supporting more weight per surface area than any other joint in the body.[32] Talar body fractures account for between 13% and 23% of all talar fractures and 0.62% of all fractures.[12,33,34] There has been a lack of clarity in differentiating between talar neck and body fractures, and this is a possible explanation for the wide range in occurrence rates of talar body fractures. Inokuchi and Ogawa[21] attempted to clarify this by using the lateral process of the talus to differentiate these fractures. Fractures in which the inferior fracture line is located anterior to the lateral process of the talus are determined to be talar neck fractures, whereas fractures located within or posterior to the lateral process of the talus are considered true talar body fractures.[21] Talar body fractures typically involve 1 or both of the ankle and subtalar joints and are therefore intra-articular fractures, making reconstruction of the talar body and maintenance of congruent articular surfaces particularly crucial.[35]

Identification and diagnosis of talar body fractures is usually done with standard radiographic images, but determination of the extent of comminution and intra-articular involvement is primarily done with additional CT images.[8] Talar body fractures are classified in multiple ways. The Sneppen classification, described by Sneppen and Christensten,[36] includes 6 parts: type A, a compression or osteochondral dome fracture; type B, a coronal shear fracture; type C, a sagittal shear fracture; type D, a posterior tubercle fracture; type E, a lateral tubercle fracture; and type F, a crush or comminuted fracture of the talus (**Box 2**).

The Fortin classification is a simpler method of classification, described by Fortin and Balazsy,[8] which includes 3 groups: type 1, a talar body fracture in any plane; type 2, a talar process or tubercle fracture; and type 3, a compression or impaction fracture of the talar body (**Box 3**).

OSTEOCHONDRAL TALAR FRACTURES

Commonly referred to as osteochondritis dissecans (OCD), transchondral dome fractures of the talus are defined as a defect in the articular cartilage, usually involving the subchondral bone.[37] These lesions were first described by Kappis[38] in 1922.[39] The terms lesion and fracture have often been used interchangeably to describe OCD. It is generally accepted that these lesions are a result of force or impact transmitted from the adjacent articulating bone or joint surface, damaging the articular cartilage and subchondral bone of the joint surface, which may initially go unrecognized by the patient.[37,40] OCD lesions account for about 1% of all talar fractures. The most widely accepted system for classifying OCD lesions was presented by Berndt and Harty[37] in 1959 and modified with an additional stage by Scranton and McDermott[41] in 2001. Stage 1 is a subchondral bone compression. Stage 2 is a partially detached osteochondral fragment. Stage 3 is a completely detached, but nondisplaced, osteochondral fragment. Stage 4 is a completely detached, displaced osteochondral fragment. Stage 5 is a large cyst below the articular surface (**Box 4**).

OCD lesions are often overlooked or misdiagnosed as ankle sprains. Clinically, initial presentation consists of a description of ankle injury, usually while participating in sports-related activities, with pain, swelling, joint stiffness, and painful range of motion. Although insignificant in appearance and difficult to diagnose, these lesions can be a significant source of pain. With the increased availability of MRI and CT imaging, as well as technetium bone scans, OCD lesions of the talus are being diagnosed more frequently (**Fig. 6**).[42]

Box 2
Sneppen classification of talar body fractures

A. Compression or osteochondral dome fracture

B. Coronal shear fracture

C. Sagittal shear fracture

D. Posterior tubercle fracture

E. Lateral tubercle fracture

F. Crush/comminuted fracture

Box 3
Fortin classification of talar body fractures

1. Talar body fractures (horizontal, sagittal, coronal, shear)

2. Talar process or tubercle fractures

3. Compression or impaction fractures

OCD lesions are typically separated into 2 categories: lateral lesions (43%) and medial lesions (56%).[37,44] The mechanism of injury, treatment, and outcomes are closely related to the location of the lesion. Medial lesions are usually less symptomatic and are commonly self-limiting in nature, attributed to medial lesions being typically deep and cup shaped.[37,43] Lateral lesions tend to be more symptomatic and rarely heal spontaneously, tending to be shallow and wafer shaped.[39] Many different mechanisms for OCD lesions have been studied, but it is widely accepted that medial lesions occur as a result of plantarflexion and inversion trauma, whereas lateral lesions occur as a result of dorsiflexion and inversion trauma.[37,43] In stable and nondisplaced OCD fragments, capillary budding can occur across the fracture line and assist in healing the defect, whereas displaced unstable fragments often undergo avascular necrosis.[37]

Treatment

General agreement on treatment of OCD lesions is based on the Berndt and Harty classification scheme. Stage 1 and 2 lesions are usually treated conservatively with activity modification and non–weight bearing with limited ankle motion via walking boot or casting. Stage 3 lesions, located medially, are most often treated with this conservative method as well, but some controversy does exist. Stage 3 lesions, located laterally, and all stage 4 lesions are recommended for surgical intervention.[31,39,43,44] Surgical intervention typically involves 1 or a combination of the following techniques: removal of loose bodies, drilling and curettage, microfracture, reduction and fixation of fragments, application of fibrin glue, osteochondral autologous transplantation, chondrocyte transplantation, and mosaicplasty.[39,40] Osteochondral autologous transplantation, chondrocyte transplantation, and mosaicplasty are usually reserved for recurring or large lesions.

TRUE BODY FRACTURES

Shear fractures of the talar body are usually the result of an axial load placed on a hyperdorsiflexed foot.[28] Sneppen and Christensten[36] made a distinction between

---

Box 4
Berndt and Harty classification of talar dome fractures

Stage 1: subchondral bone compression

Stage 2: partially detached osteochondral fragment

Stage 3: completely detached, nondisplaced osteochondral fragment

Stage 4: completely detached, displaced osteochondral fragment

Stage 5: presence of large cyst below the articular surface

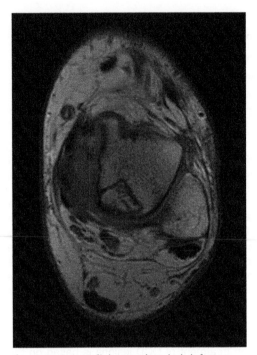

Fig. 6. An MRI scan of a posterior medial osteochondral defect.

(1) shear fractures of the medial body as a result of supination trauma, and (2) those of the lateral talar body as a result of pronation/external rotation. Falls from a height are another common mechanism of talar body fractures, in which the talus is compressed between the calcaneus and tibial plafond (**Fig. 7**). Spinal injuries should be highly suspected in this type of injury.

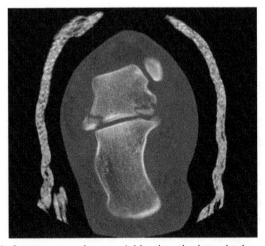

Fig. 7. A talar body fracture cause by an axial load to the lateral talus.

Sneppen and Christensten[36] concluded that the outcome of talar body fractures can be directly correlated with the severity of the initial injury, with specific emphasis on the occurrence of subluxation and associated articular damage to the talotibial and subtalar joints. They found that, in cases of compression injuries to the talar body, 50% had tibiotalar arthritis, 41% had posttraumatic arthritis of both the tibiotalar and subtalar joints, and an additional 24% had posttraumatic arthritis of either the tibiotalar or subtalar joints. Other complications associated with talar body fractures include malunion, nonunion, ankylosis, and infection.[33]

Treatment

Nondisplaced talar body fractures can be treated with 4 to 8 weeks' non–weight bearing in a short leg cast with gradual return to weight bearing.[45]

Displaced shear fractures should be repaired via open reduction and internal fixation with a goal of restoring joint integrity. Ebraheim and Patil[33] suggest that, after surgery, patients should be immobilized and non–weight bearing in a controlled ankle movement–type boot for 10 to 12 weeks with early range of motion. They suggest that additional radiography, CT, and MRI should be performed postoperatively to determine the presence of healing and the progression to weight-bearing status. In their study, approximately 50% of patients had good to excellent outcomes according to the American Orthopaedic Foot and Ankle Society rating system.[33] Comminuted talar body fractures have a worse prognosis and higher rate of complications than other talar body fractures. The risk of avascular necrosis or arthritis in comminuted fractures is estimated to be between 55% and 88% in some cases. It is suggested that patients with these types of injuries should be counseled about potential complications and their long-term outcomes.[33,35,46] The choice of surgical approach for reduction and fixation of talar body fractures is usually determined by fracture pattern and location; however, because of the difficulty in accessing the tibiotalar and subtalar joints, multiple options should be considered. Distraction of the tibiotalar joint has been performed in the past to assist with exposure, but can have additional risks in patients with acute injuries, thus medial and/or lateral malleolar osteotomies are preferred for repair.

For several weeks to months, patients with talar body fractures should be monitored and evaluated for complications.[35] The most common complication is tibiotalar arthritis, occurring in up to 65% of talar dome fractures. Subtalar arthritis can occur in as many as 35% of cases.[35] Although the risk for avascular necrosis is still present with talar body fractures (almost 38%), the risk is much less than with displaced talar neck fractures, and is most commonly seen in combination injuries that involve fractures of the talar body and dislocation of the talus from the ankle mortise and/or subtalar joints.[35,47]

LATERAL PROCESS FRACTURES

Lateral process fractures of the talus account for nearly 20% of all talar fractures.[36,48] There seems to be an increased incidence of lateral process fractures in recent years, which many investigators attribute to the increased popularity of snowboarding.[49–51] Kirkpatrick and Hunter[50] found that lateral process fractures are present in 2.3% of all snowboarding injuries, and that 34% of ankle fractures occurred while snowboarding. Chan and Yoshida[49] showed that snowboarders have a 17 times greater risk of lateral talar process fractures than nonsnowboarders. Because of this strong correlation, lateral process fractures are frequently referred to as snowboarder's fractures.[50–52]

Lateral process fractures of the talus are usually a result of a combination of dorsi-flexory and inversion forces. On inversion of the foot, the navicular shifts medially and the lateral process is moved upward on the posterior calcaneal facet, concentrating dorsiflexory forces on the lateral process, resulting in its fracture. This fracture usually presents as either a shearing or comminution fracture of the lateral process. Lateral process fractures are difficult to diagnose and commonly overlooked on initial diagnosis in emergency rooms.[48,53] Patients often present with symptoms similar to lateral ankle injuries, such as pain and swelling in the sinus tarsi. One diagnostic test to increase suspicion of a lateral process fracture rather than lateral ankle sprains is the absence of an anterior drawer sign.[7] Plain ankle films, often non–weight bearing, are usually sufficient to diagnose the injury. However, CT scans may be necessary to diagnose and determine the extent of the fracture, particularly in evaluating the extent of articular involvement (**Fig. 8**).[7,33]

The most widely accepted method of classification for lateral talar process fractures is the Hawkins classification, which is distinct from the Hawkins classification of talar neck fractures. Type 1 is a simple 2-part fracture, type 2 is a comminuted fracture of the lateral process, and type 3 is a chip fracture of the anteroinferior portion of the lateral process (**Box 5**).[48]

Treatment

Nondisplaced type 1 and 3 lateral process fractures are commonly treated without surgery with immobilization in a non–weight-bearing short leg cast for 4 to 6 weeks. Several studies have shown consistently poor outcomes for patients treated with casting alone, because of the difficulty in maintaining accurate anatomic reduction and alignment.[48,51,54,55] Patients who fail conservative casting and immobilization with continued pain and symptoms should undergo open or arthroscopic resection and remodeling of the lateral process, but this should be delayed until approximately 6 months after the initial injury.[7]

Type 2 fractures or displaced type 1 and 3 lateral process fractures are usually treated with either open reduction and internal fixation for larger fracture fragments, or excision of the fragment for smaller ones.[48,51] Excision of smaller fragments is favored by most investigators, whereas open reduction and internal fixation is recommended for larger displaced fragments.[4,54] Better outcomes have been found in patients who underwent open reduction and internal fixation or excision of fragments for displaced lateral process fractures than in those patients treated conservatively.[52]

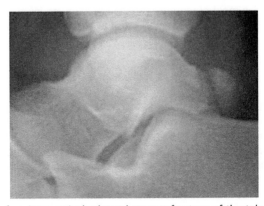

Fig. 8. A CT scan of an intra-articular lateral process fracture of the talus.

> **Box 5**
> **Hawkins classification of lateral process fractures of the talus**
>
> Type 1: simple 2-part fracture
>
> Type 2: comminuted fracture
>
> Type 3: chip fracture of anteroinferior portion

POSTERIOR PROCESS FRACTURES

Fractures of the posterior process of the talus are identified by the specific anatomic location of the fracture. Fractures of the posterolateral tubercle are frequently referred to as Shepherd fractures (**Fig. 9**).[14,56] Fractures of the posteromedial tubercle are referred to as Cedell fractures.[14,56] Shepherd fractures are more common than Cedell fractures.[14,56]

Posterior talar process fractures are often the result of forced plantarflexion of the ankle, causing compression of the process between the calcaneus and tibia.[16,57] This type of injury is often seen in athletes and dancers, especially those with frequent plantarflexed positions of the foot, such as in soccer and ballet.[58,59] Direct trauma to the posterior ankle can also be a mechanism of injury to the region. Clinically, suspicion of a posterior process fracture can be determined with a thorough description of the mechanism of injury, pain to the posterior malleolus, pain on palpation to the posterior triangle, and pain with active range of motion of the hallux as the flexor hallucis longus passes between the 2 tubercles. However, the most reliable clinical indicator is the presence of a positive nutcracker sign, which presents as pain to the area on forced plantarflexion of the ankle, named in reference to its common occurrence in ballet dancers.[28,60]

It is important to make a distinction between posterior process fractures and an accessory ossicle often located posteriorly, known as an os trigonum. Radiographically,

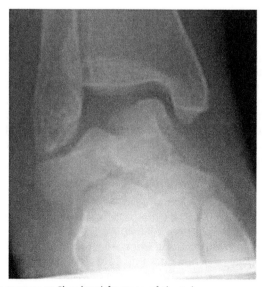

Fig. 9. A posterior process or Shepherd fracture of the talus.

the distinction can be made between a fracture, with its irregular edges, and an accessory os trigonum, which is most often round or oval with smooth well-defined edges. An os trigonum can also be identified by its presence on contralateral films. When radiographs are indeterminate, technetium bone scans may be useful in confirming the presence or absence of a fracture versus os trigonum. A negative scan negates fracture and leads to a higher suspicion of either a symptomatic os trigonum or painful inflammatory soft tissue injury.[61]

Treatment

Posterior talar process fractures are typically treated with 4 to 6 weeks of immobilization, non–weight bearing in a short leg cast, with early range of motion, and physical therapy to decrease the potential complication of flexor hallucis longus tendon adhesion.[7] Other conservative therapies include the use of nonsteroidal antiinflammatory drugs and corticosteroid injections. If conservative options fail, excision of bony fragments may be necessary.[7,62]

COMMON COMPLICATIONS IN ALL TALAR FRACTURES

Complications of talar fractures are common and can vary greatly. The worst complication, previously discussed, is avascular necrosis resulting from disrupted blood supply to the talus. Posttraumatic arthritis is the most common complication after talar fractures, seen in as many as 50% to 100% of cases.[63,64] Arthritis occurs in the talonavicular and ankle joints, but primarily affects the subtalar joint. This condition may be caused by the unique articulation and combination of compression and shearing forces between the talus and calcaneus during injury, damaging the cartilage in this joint.[65] Although arthritis is a common sequela of talar fractures, it may often be asymptomatic. Symptomatic cases of posttraumatic arthritis can be treated with a variety of conservative treatments including bracing, orthoses, ankle-foot orthoses, and activity modification. When conservative treatments fail, more aggressive options can be pursued, such as arthrodesis of the affected joint.

SUMMARY

Talar fractures can be difficult to diagnose and are complex in their nature and outcome. A thorough knowledge of the anatomy, blood supply, recommended treatments, and potential complications is necessary to optimally manage such injuries. Deciding between nonoperative versus operative treatment of talar fractures depends on the degree of displacement and comminution present. Achieving accurate anatomic reduction and ensuring that reduction is maintained via continued imaging is a vital part of treatment. Long-term outcomes, including preventing the high incidence of osteonecrosis and posttraumatic arthritis, depend on ongoing management of talar fractures and educating patients as to potential outcomes.

REFERENCES

1. Haliburton RA, Sullivan CR. The extra-osseous and intra-osseous blood supply of the talus. J Bone Joint Surg Am 1958;40:1115–20.
2. Coltart WD. Aviator's astragalus. J Bone Joint Surg Br 1952;34-B:545–66.
3. Anderson HG. The medical and surgical aspects of aviation. London: Oxford Medical Publications; 1919.
4. Adelaar RS. Complex fractures of the talus. Instr Course Lect 1997;46:323–38.

5. Mulfinger GL, Trueta J. The blood supply of the talus. J Bone Joint Surg Br 1970; 52:160–7.

6. Peterson L, Goldie I. The arterial supply of the talus: a study on the relationship to experimental talus fractures. Acta Orthop Scand 1975;46:1026–34.

7. Schuberth JM, Alder DC. Talar fractures. McGlamry's comprehensive textbook of foot and ankle surgery. 3rd edition. Philadelphia: Lippincott Williams & Wilkins; 2001.

8. Fortin PT, Balazsy JE. Talus fractures: evaluation and treatment. J Am Acad Orthop Surg 2001;9:114–27.

9. Buckley R, Sands A. Talus – multifragmentary neck fractures. Switzerland: AO Foundation; 2011. AO Surgery Reference. Available at: www.2.aofoundation. org. Accessed January 13, 2012.

10. Canale ST, Kelly FB Jr. Fractures of the neck of the talus: long-term evaluation of seventy-one cases. J Bone Joint Surg Am 1978;60:143–56.

11. Pennal GE. Fractures of the talus. Clin Orthop 1963;30:53–63.

12. Early J. Management of fractures of the talus: body and head regions. Foot Ankle Clin 2004;9:709–22.

13. Sanders R. Fractures and fracture-dislocations of the talus. In: Couglin M, Mann R, editors. Surgery of the foot and ankle. St Louis (MO): Mosby; 1999. p. 1465–518.

14. Ahmad J. Current concepts review: talar fractures. Foot Ankle Int 2006;27: 475–82.

15. Adelaar RS, Marion JR. Avascular necrosis of the talus. Orthop Clin North Am 2004;35:383–95.

16. Shishui L, Hak DJ. Management of talar neck fractures. Orthopedics 2011;34: 715–21.

17. Juliano P, Dabbah M, Harris T. Talar neck fractures. Foot Ankle Clin 2004;9: 723–36.

18. Daniels TR, Smith JW. Talar neck fractures. Foot Ankle Clin 1993;14:225–34.

19. Penny JN. Fractures and fracture dislocation of the neck of the talus. J Trauma 1980;20:1029–37.

20. Sneppen O, Buhl O. Fracture of the talus: a study of its genesis and morphology based upon cases with associated ankle fracture. Acta Orthop Scand 1974;45: 307–20.

21. Inokuchi S, Ogawa K. Classification of fractures of the talus: clear differentiation between neck and body fractures. Foot Ankle Int 1996;17:748–50.

22. Peterson L, Goldie I. Fractures of the neck of the talus: a clinical study. Acta Orthop Scand 1977;48:696–706.

23. Hawkins LG. Fractures of the neck of the talus. J Bone Joint Surg Am 1970;52: 991–1002.

24. Canale ST. Fractures of the neck of the talus. Orthopedics 1990;13:1105–15.

25. Cronier P, Talha A. Central talar fractures: therapeutic considerations. Injury 2004; 35:SB10–22.

26. Patel R, Van Bergeyk A, Pinney S. Are displaced talar neck fractures surgical emergencies? Foot Ankle Int 2005;26:378–81.

27. Berlet GC, Lee TH, Massa EG. Talar neck fractures. Orthop Clin North Am 2001; 32:53–64.

28. Thordarson D. Talar body fractures. Orthop Clin North Am 2001;32:65–77.

29. Marsh JL, Saltzman CL. Major open injuries of the talus. J Orthop Trauma 1995;9: 371–6.

30. Donnelly EF. The Hawkin's sign. Radiology 1999;210:195–6.

31. Canale ST, Beldin RH. Osteochondral lesions of the talus. J Bone Joint Surg Am 1980;62:97–102.
32. Metzger MJ, Levin JS. Talar neck fractures and rates of avascular necrosis. J Foot Ankle Surg 1999;38:154–62.
33. Ebraheim NA, Patil V. Clinical outcome of fractures of the talar body. Int Orthop 2008;32:773–7.
34. Higgins TF, Baumgartner MR. Diagnosis and treatment of fractures of the talus: a comprehensive review. Foot Ankle Int 1999;20:595–605.
35. Vallier HA, Nork SE. Surgical treatment of talar body fractures. J Bone Joint Surg Am 2003;85:1716–24.
36. Sneppen O, Christensten SB. Fracture of the body of the talus. Acta Orthop Scand 1977;48:317–24.
37. Berndt AL, Harty M. Transchondral fractures (osteochondritis dissecans) of the talus. J Bone Joint Surg Am 1959;41:988–1020.
38. Kappis M. Wietere beitrage zur traumatisch-mechanischen enstehung der "spontanen" knorpelablosungen. Dtsch Z Chir 1922;171:13 [in German].
39. Fallat LM, Morgan JH. Osteochondroses of the Foot. McGlamry's comprehensive textbook of foot and ankle surgery. 3rd edition. Philadelphia: Lippincott Williams & Wilkins; 2001. p. 2075–96.
40. Raikin SM. Stage VI: massive osteochondral defects of the talus. Foot Ankle Clin 2004;9:737–44.
41. Scranton PE Jr, McDermott JE. Treatment of type V osteochondral lesions of the talus with ipsilateral knee osteochondral autografts. Foot Ankle Int 2001;22:380–4.
42. Scharling M. Osteochondritis dissecans of the talus. Acta Orthop Scand 1978;49:89–94.
43. Flick AB, Gould N. Osteochondritis dissecans of the talus: review of the literature and new surgical approach for medial dome lesions. Foot Ankle 1985;5:165–85.
44. Pettine KA, Morrey BF. Osteochondral fractures of the talus – a long term follow-up. J Bone Joint Surg Br 1987;69:89–92.
45. Mindell ER, Cisek EE. Late results of injuries to the talus: analysis of forty cases. J Bone Joint Surg Am 1963;45:221–45.
46. Cantrell M, Tarquinio T. Fracture of the lateral process of the talus. Orthopedics 2000;23:55–8.
47. Kleiger B, Ahmed M. Injuries of the talus and its joints. Clin Orthop 1976;121:243–62.
48. Hawkins LG. Fracture of the lateral process of the talus. J Bone Joint Surg Am 1965;47:1170–5.
49. Chan GM, Yoshida D. Fracture of the lateral process of the talus associated with snowboarding. Ann Emerg Med 2003;41:854–8.
50. Kirkpatrick DP, Hunter RE. The snowboarder's foot and ankle. Am J Sports Med 1998;26:271–7.
51. Heckman J, Maclean M. Fractures of the lateral process of the talus. Clin Orthop 1985;199:108–13.
52. Valderrabano V, Perren T. Snowboarder's talus fracture: treatment outcome of 20 cases after 3.5 years. Am J Sports Med 2005;33:871–80.
53. Mukherjee SK, Pringle RM. Fracture of the lateral process of the talus: a report of thirteen cases. J Bone Joint Surg Br 1974;56:263–73.
54. Dimon JH. Isolated displaced fractures of the posterior facet of the talus. J Bone Joint Surg Am 1961;43:275–81.
55. Vallier HA, Nork SE. Talar neck fractures: results and outcomes. J Bone Joint Surg Am 2004;86:1616–24.

56. Cedell CA. Rupture of the posterior talotibial ligament with avulsion of a bone fragment from the talus. Acta Orthop Scand 1974;45:454–61.
57. Hedrick MR, McBryde AM. Posterior ankle impingement. Foot Ankle Int 1994;15: 2–8.
58. Kleiger B. Fractures of the talus. J Bone Joint Surg Am 1948;30:735–44.
59. Paulos LE, Johnson CL. Posterior compartment fractures of the ankle: a commonly missed athletic injury. Am J Sports Med 1983;11:439–43.
60. Fricker PA, Williams JG. Surgical management of os trigonum and talar spur in sportsmen. Br J Sports Med 1979;13:55–7.
61. Johnson RP, Collier BD. The os trigonum syndrome: use of bone scan in the diagnosis. J Trauma 1984;24:761–4.
62. Marotta JJ, Micheli LJ. Os trigonum impingement in dancers. Am J Sports Med 1992;20:533–6.
63. Frawley PA, Hart JA. Treatment outcome of major fractures of the talus. Foot Ankle Int 1995;16:339–45.
64. Lindvall E, Haidukewych G. Open reduction and stable fixation of isolated displaced talar neck and body fractures. J Bone Joint Surg Am 2004;86:2229–34.
65. Saltsman C, Marsh JL. Hindfoot dislocations: when are they not benign? J Am Acad Orthop Surg 1997;5:192–8.

Calcaneal Fractures: Update on Current Treatments

Kathie Palmersheim, BS[a], Blake Hines, BA[a], Ben L. Olsen, DPM[b,*]

KEYWORDS

• Calcaneal fractures • Current treatment • Update

Calcaneal fractures represent 2% of all fractures and account for approximately 60% of all tarsal injuries.[1,2] Historically, it has been understood that these fractures are debilitating and are likely to involve extensive complications.[3] Motor vehicle collisions and falls from a height are the major causes of these large force compression injuries, causing widening of the heel, loss of heel height, and large amounts of articular surface displacement.[1] A strong correlation has been shown between restoration of normal anatomy and satisfactory functional outcome.[4] It is necessary to be familiar with the basic fundamentals of calcaneal fractures, including the anatomy, the radiographic findings, and the challenges that these complicated fractures present. Once these principles are understood, the physician can then be ready with the armamentarium that allows for a patient-specific and injury-specific plan.

OSSEOUS ANATOMY

Recognizing the landmarks and characteristics of the calcaneus is paramount when assessing the extent of a calcaneal injury. This tarsal bone comprises 6 different surfaces and 4 articular facets. The most anterior facet articulates with the cuboid bone, forming the calcaneal-cuboid joint. Superiorly, the anterior, middle, and posterior facets articulate with the talus, forming the subtalar joint. On the medial aspect of the calcaneus is the sustentaculum tali. This eminence supports the middle articular facet, with the extrinsic foot flexors and neurovascular bundle passing beneath it. Along the lateral side of the calcaneus is the trochlear process, with an inferior groove for the peroneus longus tendon.[5]

The calcaneus consists of cancellous bone surrounded by a thin cortical shell. The cortical shell is of a higher density where it underlies the subtalar facets and is referred to as thalamic bone. The thalamic bone allows for increased axial loads along the

Disclosure: Primary author has been a paid consultant for Tornier Medical.
[a] Department of Foot and Ankle Surgery, Des Moines University, 3200 Grand Avenue, Des Moines, IA 50312, USA
[b] Department of Foot and Ankle Surgery, Broadlawns Medical Center, Des Moines, IA 50314, USA
* Corresponding author.
E-mail address: bolsen@broadlawns.org

Clin Podiatr Med Surg 29 (2012) 205–220
doi:10.1016/j.cpm.2012.01.007
0891-8422/12/$ – see front matter © 2012 Elsevier Inc. All rights reserved.

angle of Gissane. This angle is formed by the intersection of the downward and upward slopes of the superior calcaneal surface and is located directly inferior to the lateral process of the talus.[6] Within the cancellous bone, traction and compression trabeculae are formed, which allow for accommodation of axial and sheer stresses during ambulation. Where these patterns come together below the thalamic bone of the subtalar joint, there is an area where the trabeculae are sparse, termed the neutral triangle. This area is considered the weakest part of the bone and consequently most fractures usually occur there.[5,6]

RADIOGRAPHIC EVALUATION

Classifications and radiographic features of calcaneal fractures must be understood before proper evaluation can be performed. Essex-Lopresti[7] divides calcaneal fractures into tongue-type and joint-depression-type fractures based on plain film radiographic evaluation. In the tongue-type fracture, the primary fracture lines exit the calcaneus through the posterior tuberosity, and the posterior facet remains attached to this superior fragment. This situation makes it possible to position the posterior facet through manipulation of this fragment. In the joint-depression-type fracture, the primary fracture line exits superiorly behind the posterior facet, creating a fragment separate from the posterior tubercle. Rowe and colleagues[8] developed a classification system describing these fractures as: "Type 1A–fracture of tuberosity; 1B–fracture of sustentaculum tali; 1C–fracture of anterior process; 2A–beak fracture; 2B–avulsion fracture of insertion of Achilles tendon; 3A/B–oblique fracture not involving sub-talar joint; 4A/B–fracture involving sub-talar joint; 5A/B–central depression fracture with comminution." The primary classification currently used in evaluation of calcaneal fractures was described by Sanders and colleagues,[9] in 1993, based on computed tomography (CT). Sanders and colleagues described calcaneal fractures based on the fracture line(s) through the posterior facet visible on a coronal view: type 1, nondisplaced; type 2, displaced with the posterior facet in 2 fragments (with A, B, and C after the number to denote fracture location(s)); type 3, with the posterior facet having 3 major fracture fragments (also with accompanying letter for fracture locations); and type 4, comminuted (**Fig. 1**).

Bohler's is the most recognized and accepted radiographic parameter visible on a lateral plain film radiograph. The Bohler angle is measured at the intersection of lines drawn from the anterior tuberosity of the calcaneus to the most dorsal point of the posterior facet and from the posterior facet to the posterior tuberosity.[10] The normal range for the Bohler angle is 25° to 40°; a vertical compression fracture of the calcaneus causes a decrease or flattening of this angle (**Figs. 2 and 3**).

CHALLENGES

Calcaneal fractures typically represent high-energy injuries associated with significant soft tissue compromise.[11] Coexistent traumatic injury must be considered. Common injuries to suspect include contralateral calcaneal fractures, ankle fractures, vertebral (especially L1) fractures, femoral, wrist, and other tarsal bone fractures.[5] In cases of significant trauma, it is important to perform a full workup, focusing on the liver, spleen, and bladder.

High-energy calcaneal fractures lead to intense edema, a devastating development in an area with such a fragile soft tissue envelope, which causes delay in treatment, fracture blisters, and compartment syndrome. It is therefore essential to respect the soft tissue and focus on its management from the start, thus improving healing and decreasing wound complications.[11]

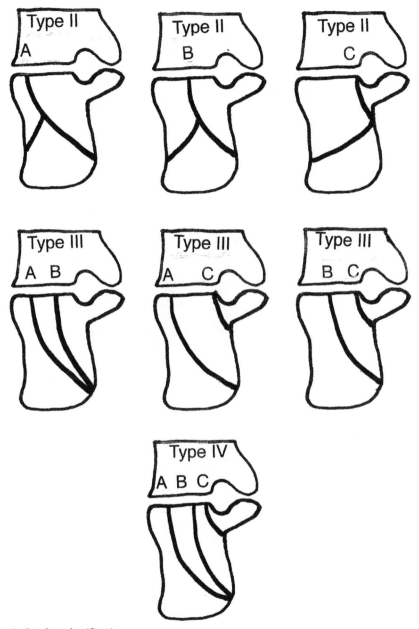

Fig. 1. Sanders classification.

Surgical correction is ideally carried out within 6 to 8 hours of injury.[5] If this correction cannot be accomplished, delaying surgery to allow time for the swelling to subside is a widely accepted practice in calcaneal fracture repair. Reducing the edema minimizes complications related to wound healing and produces better results.[12] After injury, 7 to 14 days are recommended for reduction of edema. Toward this end, compression, ice, elevation, and immobilization should be practiced before surgery.[2] Return of normal skin wrinkles is an indication that edema has subsided enough for operative intervention.

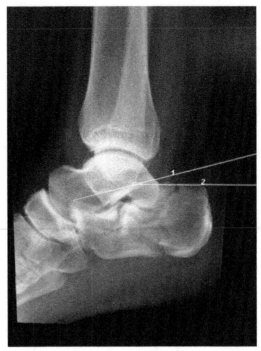

Fig. 2. Calcaneal fracture with depressed posterior facet of the subtalar joint showing decrease in Bohler angle.

Surgery should not be delayed more than 2 weeks, because subsequent fibrosis between fragments decreases their mobility, thus increasing surgical difficulty.[13]

Fracture blisters are another preoperative challenge in high-energy fractures. Management of these blisters is still controversial. Fracture blisters are hypothesized to result from large strains applied to the skin during the initial fracture deformation, causing a cleavage injury at the dermoepidermal junction. These injuries most often occur at sites where skin is closely adhered to bone and there is no muscle or enveloping fascia present.[14] On the patient's admittance to hospital, compression, ice, and elevation are required to prevent blisters from occurring.[4] If already present, blisters can be allowed to resolve before surgery, or they can be ignored and cut through during surgery. Moist antibiotic dressings are then used to prevent superficial wound infection after surgery.[5]

Because of the high-energy mechanism, bony morphology of the calcaneus, and usual comminution of these fractures, compartment syndrome can be a complicating factor. Manoli and Weber[15] identified 9 compartments in the foot. The compartment with the highest pressures and greatest potential for this complication is the calcaneal compartment, consisting of the quadratus plantae muscle, the lateral plantar nerve, and occasionally the medial plantar nerve.[5] During fracture, the calcaneal compartment pressures can increase drastically, leading to compartment syndrome. It was originally believed that approximately 10% of patients with these fractures developed compartment syndrome of the foot, with half of these leading to clawing of the toes and other toe deformities.[16] In Howard and colleagues', prospective randomized study,[17] only 6 of 459 (1%) developed compartment syndrome, suggesting that this complication may not be as common as was once believed. Diagnosis of compartment syndrome begins

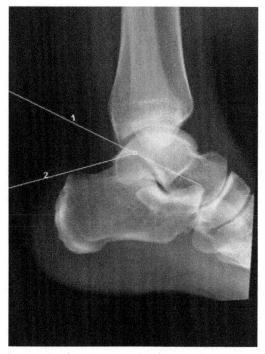

Fig. 3. Contralateral extremity showing normal Bohler angle.

with a heightened level of clinical suspicion based on the mechanism of injury. The primary indication of evolving compartment syndrome is pain out of proportion to the injury. This pain is exacerbated with passive dorsiflexion of the toes, which stretches the intrinsic musculature of the foot.[18] An absent pulse or complete anesthesia are late findings in compartment syndrome, and may be difficult to diagnose under circumstances of massive swelling. The only objective method to diagnose compartment syndrome is to measure the absolute compartment pressures.[18] Most institutions use a simple intracompartmental pressure monitoring system. To measure the calcaneal compartment pressure the needle is inserted 5 cm distal and 2 cm inferior to the medial malleolus. The needle is advanced through the abductor hallucis, and directed inferiorly toward the posterior tuberosity of the calcaneus.[18] If the compartment pressure exceeds 30 mm Hg, or if compartment pressure is less than 10 to 30 mm Hg less than diastolic pressure, fasciotomy is indicated.[19] The approaches for calcaneal compartment decompression generally include a medial incision over the compartment. If further decompression is needed in the forefoot, 2 longitudinal incisions can be made dorsally.[19] The wounds are left open for 5 to 7 days, followed by delayed primary closure or split-thickness skin graft.[5,19] The consequences of untreated compartment syndrome of the foot include clawing of the lesser toes, stiffness, chronic pain, motor weakness, neurovascular dysfunction, and fixed deformities of the foot.[16]

APPROACH AND FIXATION
Fracture Treatment

Understanding of the anatomy and fracture patterns has progressed along with the development of advanced surgical techniques, so current treatment protocol has shifted toward open reduction and internal fixation. Closed reduction and nonoperative treatment are being used only in specific cases. When determining the appropriate approach, several factors are considered: age, health, gender, mechanism of injury, soft tissue integrity, comminution, and Bohler angle.[20] Of these variables, several investigators have found Bohler angle to be the primary determining factor of outcome. Regardless of surgical or nonsurgical treatment, significantly better outcomes result from restoration of the Bohler angle to its original value and reconstruction of the subtalar joint surface.[1,21] After a 6.5-year follow-up of a previous study, Paul and colleagues[22] determined that a Bohler angle of less than 10° was associated with poor outcomes if treated operatively. The results were even worse if treated nonoperatively, with increasing levels of pain and a high correlation with subtalar arthrodesis. Age and activity levels are also important considerations. Nonoperative treatment should always be considered for elderly patients who have low physical demand or major medical comorbidities that predispose them to surgical complications.[21]

Studies have found that patients undergoing operative treatment scored higher on the American Orthopaedic Foot and Ankle Society hindfoot and ankle score and the 100-mm visual analog scale pain score when compared with patients undergoing nonsurgical treatment, supporting operative treatment of improved outcomes in displaced intra-articular calcaneal fractures.[21] The goal of operative treatment is to obtain anatomic reduction of articular surfaces and restore the architecture of the nonarticular portions, minimizing wound healing complications.[23] Various factors affect the development of complications in calcaneal fractures, so it is important to tailor treatment strategy on a case-by-case basis.[17]

Percutaneous Approach

Forgona and Zadravecz's technique for closed reduction and percutaneous screw fixation was originally introduced in 1983. By using this less invasive technique, they were able to avoid many of the soft tissue complications seen in previous approaches. Tomesen and colleagues[24] modified that technique, finding a high degree of patient satisfaction in fractures with minimal comminution, tongue-type fractures, and joint-depression-type fractures. This technique works best in fracture patterns with large tuberosity and sustentaculum fragments, which provide support for the screws. Ideally, this technique is used in lower-energy fractures, in which treatment can begin shortly after initial injury. Fracture fragments are more easily manipulated during early stages of the injury. Several variations to Forgona and Zadravecz's percutaneous reduction have been studied, with each reporting consistent results. Closed reduction and percutaneous screw fixation has resulted in good patient outcomes based on quality of fracture reduction. The main complication with this technique is screw head irritation. About half required screw removal, which prevented future complications.

Plating Options

Typically in calcaneal fractures, a certain degree of comminution is present. Comminuted fractures rarely respond well to isolated screw fixation, so plate fixation has become the fixation of choice for most surgeons. Plates can be described as locking, nonlocking, or a mixture of the 2. Nonlocking plates allow compression of the plate to the bone surface, but lack a union between the screw and plate, with greater risk of screw loosening and subsequent pullout. Locking screws eliminate risk of the screw loosening from the plate, because the head of the screw is threaded to match the threaded hole of the plate. This feature reduces compression, but creates a more stable fixed-angle device.[25] Hyer and colleagues[25] have described a shorter nonweight-bearing period with a locking plate (average 4.88 weeks) compared with nonlocking plates (average 9 weeks nonweight-bearing). Radiographic evaluation also showed no significant loss of correction with locking plates. This study shows a benefit to locking plates in calcaneal fracture. However, most studies have shown that although locking plates have higher load to failure performance and greater stability with cyclic loading, no statistical difference has been shown in their use over nonlocking plates.[26–29] A study evaluating different locking plates[30] suggested that there may be benefit to using polyaxial locked versus uniaxial locked screws. This increased stability may be caused by fixation of the sustentacular fragment through the plate using the polyaxial screw.

Extended Lateral Approach

Historically, many different surgical approaches have been described in the literature for open reduction and internal fixation of calcaneal fractures.[31] Consensus is that the best visualization and restoration of the subtalar joint is through the extensile lateral approach, yet complications can arise with wound healing and nerve compromise. This hockey-stick-shaped incision is used to visualize the lateral wall of the calcaneus, the subtalar joint, and the calcaneocuboid joint (**Figs. 4** and **5**).[2] This wide exposure allows placement of a lateral plate, and lag screw fixation permits reduction of the body fragment medially. For this approach, a full-thickness lateral calcaneal flap needs to be created without disrupting the blood supply from the lateral calcaneal artery.[23] The lateral calcaneal artery has been found to supply most of the vascular supply to the corner of the flap of the extensile lateral incision, and the posterior vertical portion of the incision places this artery at risk.[32] Excessive tension or manipulation of the flap must also be avoided, because it can be detrimental to the vascularity to the tissue.[2] Complications are more common in open calcaneal fractures, smokers, and patients with diabetes.[4] In order of decreasing frequency, these complications include wound dehiscence, peroneal tendonitis, sural nerve injury, infection (requiring free flap for wound coverage), and amputation (see **Fig. 5**).[33]

Sinus Tarsi Approach

The sinus tarsi approach, or a modification of this type of incision, has been described in the literature, although less commonly than the extensile lateral approach.[4,23,31,33–38]

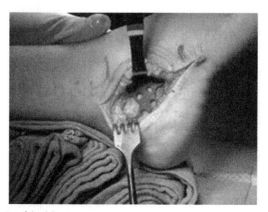

Fig. 4. Extended lateral incision.

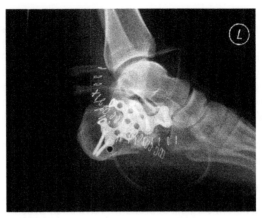

Fig. 5. Lateral calcaneal plate.

The typical incision in this technique starts 1 to 1.5 cm distal to the fibula and extends 5 to 6 cm distally to the base of the fourth metatarsal (**Fig. 6**).[33,34]

Direct exposure of the subtalar joint is achieved through this technique without the need for a large incision. The excellent visualization of the posterior subtalar and calcaneocuboid joints allows for consistent reduction of posterior subtalar joint depression and calcaneocuboid articular malalignment.[33] Because less dissection is required with this technique, it allows for shorter operating times and lessens injury to the lateral calcaneal artery.[23] Visualization is limited with this approach, and a displaced posterior tuberosity may be more difficult to reduce.[33] Postoperative CT examination showed improved posterior facet position, calcaneal height, and calcaneal width from open reduction with this technique.[33] In a systematic review of 8 case series reporting on 271 calcaneal fractures repaired using the sinus tarsi approach, fewer wound complications and sural nerve injuries were found when compared with the extensile lateral approach.[31] No standardized fixation was used in these different reports, so fixation varied from pins to screws to plates. Bone grafting or bone graft substitutes were used variably.[4,23,31,33–38] As this incision has increased in popularity, commercially available plates have been specifically designed for use with this minimal incision. We use 2 medical device companies for these types of

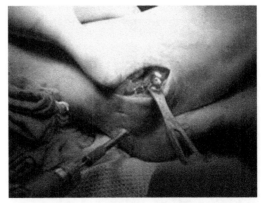

Fig. 6. Sinus tarsi incision with use of a Tornier WAVE plate and placement of a screw into the posterior arm of the plate through a minimal incision.

plates: Tornier has a stainless steel plate that they have branded the WAVE plate (Tornier, Inc., Edina, MN, USA), and Acumed has a titanium calcaneal plating system that includes specialized plates referred to as MINI-Calc plates (Acumed USA, Hillsboro, OR, USA). Both systems use locking screw technology. The Tornier system also includes an apical hole that is nonlocking, designed for use with a lag screw (**Figs. 7** and **8**).[39,40]

Circular Ring Fixation

In cases of comminution or extensive soft tissue compromise, external fixation may be indicated. Talarico and colleagues[41] retrospectively analyzed 25 intra-articular calcaneal fractures that were treated with external ring fixation at Middle Georgia Hospital. They describe a Steinmann pin driven transversely through the most posterior and plantar aspect of the calcaneus and traction applied in the sagittal plane to achieve reduction of the calcaneus. Two tibial rings and 1 foot plate were used. A small incision was made inferior to the lateral malleolus to allow for manipulation of the fracture fragments under fluoroscopic guidance. A synthetic bone graft was mixed with the patient's blood and was used to fill the void after distraction and reapproximation of the bone. Wires through the tibia and calcaneus were secured to the frame, and distraction of the subtalar joint was performed at later visits to protect the healing posterior facet of the calcaneus. Patients were able to ambulate immediately, as tolerated, with a walker. External bone stimulators were used to increase healing potential. Talarico described "good" to "excellent" outcomes in 23 of the 25 corrections at final follow-up. Some benefits of external fixation are early weight bearing, adequate distraction with severe comminution or soft tissue damage, and consistent distraction of the calcaneus at the subtalar joint while the frame is in place. Common complications associated with external fixation are pin tract infections, hardware failure, neurovascular injury and premature weight bearing (if this is not desired).

Delta Frame Fixation

Delta frame–type constructs are an alternative to open reduction or external ring fixation. It has been suggested that through this type of construct, reduction of subtalar joint depression can be accomplished through ligamentotaxis. Three pins are placed by fluoroscopy; the first in the tibia approximately 7 cm above the ankle joint, the second in the tuberosity fragment of the calcaneus, and the third through the neck of the talus. Rods then connect the tibial pin to the calcaneal pin, the tibial pin to

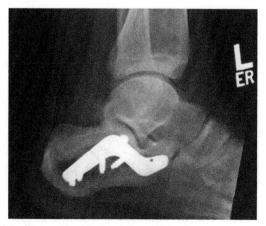

Fig. 7. Tornier WAVE plate used with the sinus tarsi incision.

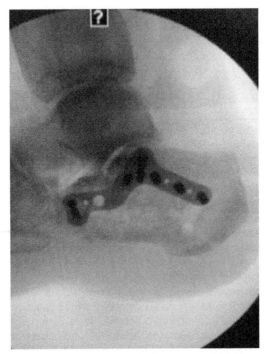

Fig. 8. Acumed MINI-Calc plate placed through the sinus tarsi incision.

the talar pin, and the talar pin to the calcaneal pin on both the medial and lateral aspects of the affected limb. Axial distraction is first performed, followed by medial and lateral distraction for proper reduction. This construct allows distraction in all 3 cardinal planes. Delta frames are contraindicated with severe comminution of the calcaneal tuberosity or fracture of the talus (**Fig. 9**).[42]

Calcaneoplasty

A new approach to managing depressed posterior calcaneal facet fractures is by calcaneoplasty. Gupta and colleagues[43] conducted a study in which percutaneous

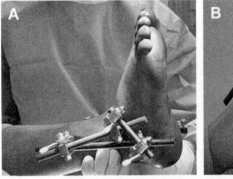
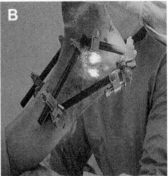

Fig. 9. Delta frame construction. (*From* Kissel CG, Husain ZS, Cottom JM, et al. Early clinical and radiographic outcomes after treatment of displaced intra-articular calcaneal fractures using delta-frame external fixator construct. J Foot Ankle Surg 2011;50:137; with permission.)

balloon reduction (traditionally used for vertebral compression fractures) was used in cases in which the varus angulation of the calcaneus was less than 5°. The procedure involves a minimal incision, with a trochar from the balloon reduction system placed fluoroscopically. The balloon is inflated slowly to achieve reduction and then rapidly inflated beyond its rupture point, and synthetic bone graft injected through the trochar. The investigators postulate that this process can eliminate the need for internal fixation and also decrease complications associated with an extensile approach.

Arthrodesis

Primary subtalar joint arthrodesis has been advocated for calcaneal fracture patterns involving extensive comminution at the posterior facet. Extensive can be defined as 4-part or more fractures.[44,45] According to Sanders and colleagues,[9,44] the rates of secondary surgical subtalar fusion may be as high as 73% in type 4 fractures; therefore, they recommend open reduction and primary subtalar arthrodesis. Other cases in which a primary subtalar joint arthrodesis is indicated are poor soft tissue envelope, open fracture, late resolution of soft tissue edema, or when the severity of the cartilage damage may lead to posttraumatic arthritis. Primary subtalar joint arthrodesis can provide better stability than isolated open reduction with internal fixation (ORIF) in patients with multiple comorbidities, including diabetes, peripheral neuropathy, and obesity.[44] The arthrodesis provides stable reduction of the deformity and prevents further collapse. Its limited incision helps to decrease wound complications in high-risk patients.[45] Treatment can be combined with an external fixation device to allow maximum stability with nonweight-bearing activity.[45]

BONE GRAFTING

Whether bone grafting is necessary in repairing calcaneal fractures is controversial.[12] In a direct comparison of displaced intra-articular calcaneal fractures,[46] no radiographic or functional benefit was found with the use of bone grafting, although the investigators do comment that resorbable bone graft substitutes may be useful to maintain the Bohler angle. When bone graft is indicated, several options are available. One of the more important questions is whether to use autogenous or allogenic bone graft material. Pollard and Schuberth[47] cited no difference in union rate with the use of autogenous and allogenic bone graft when used with arthrodesis. Lee and Talarico[48] cite the potential benefits of allogenic bone graft to be primarily associated with reduced morbidity associated with harvest of autogenous graft. They list "hemorrhage, fracture, pain, and nerve damage" as some of the avoidable complications. The use of allogenic bone graft also reduces operating time and eliminates the worry over graft compromise or inadequate void filling, because additional grafts are readily available.

Orthobiologics are becoming increasingly prevalent in treatment of fractures.[12] There are many commercially available bone graft substitutes.[49] The surgeon must take into account the composition of each product and match this to the application. Because of the cancellous nature of calcaneal bone, graft may not be necessary to promote regeneration of bone; however, the augmentation allows the defect to be filled and offers additional support of the depressed posterior facet.[12]

Closure Assistance

Another technological advancement is the use of negative pressure wound therapy (NPWT). Commonly used after wound dehiscence, it is less commonly known for its use in preventing wound dehiscence and necrosis or aiding in healing by primary intention. Stannard and colleagues[50] studied the use of NPWT in augmenting the healing of surgical incisions and the resolution of postoperative hematomas after high-energy trauma. They determined that NPWT aided in the removal of blood and excess serous fluid, preventing hematomas and wound dehiscence and therefore enhancing healing. It is also believed that the removal of interstitial fluid is important, because it contains inflammatory and potentially infectious exudate that could impair healing.[51] Use of NPWT postoperatively has also been found to decrease pain, swelling, and healing time in patients.[51] When it comes to open, high-energy fractures as well as low-energy trauma, NPWT in the immediate postoperative period is a safe, cost-effective, and viable adjunctive treatment that may decrease postoperative wound complications (**Fig. 10**).[50,51]

Secondary Complications

Complications often occur after calcaneal fractures, even when appropriate treatment has been offered. Informing the patient of potential complications, as well as recognizing variables leading up to them, is paramount to the success of the treatment. Wound-related complications can be classified as superficial or deep infections. Superficial skin infections occur in 16% of ORIF cases. These infections are usually treated on an outpatient basis with dressing changes, whirlpool, and antibiotics.[17] The extent of cellulitis, lymphangitis, or systemic signs dictates whether the infection is more serious.[52] Deep infections require hospitalization, intravenous antibiotics, debridement, and often removal of hardware or bone. Deep infections occur in 5% of ORIF cases and can cause significant morbidity for the patient.[17] The management goal for these infections is to prevent direct extension to bone causing osteomyelitis.[52] With open calcaneal fractures, overall infection rate has been found to be as high as 37%.[53] Type 3 open fractures not only have a high risk of infection, but the risk of developing osteomyelitis after treatment reaches 27% and greater. By performing early irrigation, debridement, and stabilization, astute clinicians can prevent this complication rate from increasing.[17]

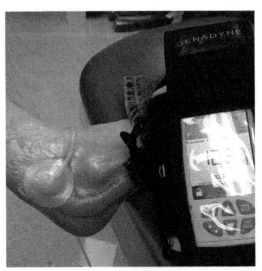

Fig. 10. Genadyne (Genadyne Biotechnologies Inc., Great Neck, NY, USA) NPWT used to assist wound healing with the lateral extensile incision.

The most common complication for both nonoperatively and operatively treated calcaneal fractures is the need for eventual or delayed surgery. For patients undergoing surgical treatment, the most common subsequent operation is for removal of hardware.[17] These procedures are usually performed to relieve pain presumed to be secondary to the hardware. Howard and colleagues[17] determined that hardware removal improved patient symptoms in each situation in their study. With nonsurgical treatment, later subtalar arthrodesis becomes more common.[17,21,45] Secondary arthrodesis is indicated after initial conservative treatment in approximately 21% to 30% of cases versus 2% to 5% of cases after operative treatment.[54] A relationship has been found between delayed healing and revision surgery, as well as between the amount of avascular subchondral bone at the subtalar joint and revision surgery.[54] Whether a secondary arthrodesis results in improved outcome after initial operative treatment, or after initial conservative treatment, remains unclear.[54] Schepers and colleagues[54] determined that there is no statistical difference between performing a secondary subtalar joint arthrodesis versus performing a secondary triple arthrodesis as therapy for symptomatic arthrosis after previously treated intra-articular calcaneal fracture.

Loss of fixation, malunion/nonunion, and overcorrection/undercorrection are also complications seen with calcaneal fracture repair. Loss of fixation and malalignment can be prevented with intraoperative fluoroscopy, although patient compliance also plays a role in maintaining fixation.[52]

SUMMARY

Through a comprehensive review of the current literature, the basics of calcaneal fractures along with several evolving techniques for calcaneal fracture treatment have been highlighted. The importance of these studies and the proper management of these fractures is not to be underestimated. In such a controversial and potentially detrimental injury, the focus on evidence-based medicine is driving treatment toward more positive patient outcomes. Through methods such as advanced imaging techniques, less invasive surgical procedures, and better postoperative care, proper strategies for care can be based on individual patient requirements.

REFERENCES

1. Molloy AP, Lipscombe SJ. Hindfoot arthrodesis for management of bone loss following calcaneus fractures and nonunions. Foot Ankle Clin 2011;16(1):165–79.
2. Hollawell S. Wound closure technique for lateral extensile approach to intra-articular calcaneal fractures. J Am Podiatr Med Assoc 2008;98(5):422–5.
3. Zwipp H, Tscherne H, Thermann H, et al. Osteosynthesis of displaced intraarticular fractures of the calcaneus. Clin Orthop Relat Res 1993;290:76–86.
4. Mostafa MF, El-Adl G, Hassanin EY, et al. Surgical treatment of displaced intra-articular calcaneal fracture using a single small lateral approach. Strategies Trauma Limb Reconstr 2010;5(2):87–95.
5. Buddecke DE Jr, Mandracchia VJ. Calcaneal fractures. Clin Podiatr Med Surg 1999;16(4):769–91.
6. Badillo K, Pacheco JA, Padua SO, et al. Multidetector CT evaluation of calcaneal fractures. Radiographics 2011;31(1):81–92.
7. Essex-Lopresti P. The mechanism, reduction technique, and results in fractures of the os calcis. Br J Surg 1952;39(157):395–419.
8. Rowe CR, Sakellarides HT, Freeman PA. Fractures of the os calcis: a long-term follow-up study of 146 patients. JAMA 1963;184:920.

9. Sanders R, Fortin P, DiPasquale T, et al. Operative treatment in 120 displaced in-traarticular calcaneal fractures. Results using a prognostic computed tomography scan classification. Clin Orthop Relat Res 1993;290:87–95.

10. Bohler L. Diagnosis, pathology and treatment of fractures of the os calcis. J Bone Joint Surg 1931;31:75.

11. Mehta S, Mirza AJ, Dunbar RP, et al. A staged treatment plan for the management of Type II and Type IIIA open calcaneus fractures. J Orthop Trauma 2010;24(3):142–7.

12. Dhillon MS, Bali K, Prabhakar S. Controversies in calcaneus fracture management: a systematic review of the literature. Musculoskelet Surg 2011;95(3):171–81.

13. Tennent TD, Calder PR, Salisbury RD, et al. The operative management of displaced intra-articular fractures of the calcaneum: a two-centre study using a defined protocol. Injury 2001;32(6):491–6.

14. Uebbing CM, Walsh M, Miller JB, et al. Fracture blisters. West J Emerg Med 2011; 12(1):131–3.

15. Manoli A 2nd, Weber TG. Fasciotomy of the foot: an anatomical study with special reference to release of the calcaneal compartment. Foot Ankle 1990;10(5): 267–75.

16. Kalsi R, Dempsey A, Bunney EB. Compartment syndrome of the foot after calcaneal fracture. J Emerg Med 2009;8:59.

17. Howard JL, Buckley R, McCormack R, et al. Complications following management of displaced intra-articular calcaneal fractures: a prospective randomized trial comparing open reduction internal fixation with nonoperative management. J Orthop Trauma 2003;17(4):241–9.

18. Haddad SL. Managing risk: compartment syndromes of the foot. AAOS Now 2007;1(1).

19. Fulkerson E, Razi A, Tejwani N. Review: acute compartment syndrome of the foot. Foot Ankle Int 2003;24(2):180–7.

20. Dooley P, Buckley R, Tough S, et al. Bilateral calcaneal fractures: operative versus nonoperative treatment. Foot Ankle Int 2004;25(2):47–52.

21. Basile A. Operative versus nonoperative treatment of displaced intra-articular calcaneal fractures in elderly patients. J Foot Ankle Surg 2010;49(1):25–32.

22. Paul M, Peter R, Hoffmeyer P. Fractures of the calcaneum. A review of 70 patients. J Bone Joint Surg Br 2004;86(8):1142–5.

23. Femino JE, Vaseenon T, Levin DA, et al. Modification of the sinus tarsi approach for open reduction and plate fixation of intra-articular calcaneus fractures: the limits of proximal extension based upon the vascular anatomy of the lateral calcaneal artery. Iowa Orthop J 2010;30:161–7.

24. Tomesen T, Biert J, Frolke JP. Treatment of displaced intra-articular calcaneal fractures with closed reduction and percutaneous screw fixation. J Bone Joint Surg Am 2011;93(10):920–8.

25. Hyer CF, Atway S, Berlet GC, et al. Early weight bearing of calcaneal fractures fixated with locked plates: a radiographic review. Foot Ankle Spec 2010;3(6): 320–3.

26. Illert T, Rammelt S. Stability of locking and non-locking plates in an osteoporotic calcaneal fracture model. Foot Ankle Int 2011;32(3):307–13.

27. Stoffel K, Booth G, Rohrl S, et al. A comparison of conventional versus locking plates in intraarticular calcaneus fractures: a biomechanical study in human cadavers. Clin Biomech 2007;22:100–5.

28. Redfern D, Oliveira M, Campbell J, et al. A biomechanical comparison of locking and nonlocking plates for the fixation of calcaneal fractures. Foot Ankle Int 2006; 27(3):196–201.

29. Richter M, Gosling T, Zech S, et al. A comparison of plates with and without locking screws in a calcaneal fracture model. Foot Ankle Int 2005;26:309–19.
30. Richter M, Droste P, Goesling T, et al. Polyaxially-locked plate screws increase stability of fracture fixation in an experimental model of calcaneal fracture. J Bone Joint Surg Br 2006;88(9):1257–63.
31. Schepers T. The sinus tarsi approach in displaced intra-articular calcaneal fractures: a systematic review. Int Orthop 2011;35:697–703.
32. Borrelli J, Lashgari C. Vascularity of the lateral calcaneal flap: a cadaveric injection study. J Orthop Trauma 1999;13(73):77.
33. Gupta A, Ghalambor N, Nihal A, et al. The modified Palmer lateral approach for calcaneal fractures: wound healing and postoperative computed tomographic evaluation of fracture reduction. Foot Ankle Int 2003;24(10):744–53.
34. Hospodar P, Guzman C, Johnson P, et al. Treatment of displaced calcaneus fractures using a minimally invasive sinus tarsi approach. Orthopedics 2008;31(11): 1112.
35. Ebraheim NA, Elgafy H, Sabry FF, et al. Sinus tarsi approach with trans-articular fixation for displaced intra-articular fractures of the calcaneus. Foot Ankle Int 2000;21(2):105.
36. Geel CW, Flemister AS. Standardized treatment of intra-articular calcaneal fractures using an oblique lateral incision and no bone graft. J Trauma 2001;50(6): 1083.
37. Weber M, Lehman O, Sagesser D, et al. Limited open reduction and internal fixation of displaced intra-articular fractures of the calcaneum. J Bone Joint Surg Br 2008;90(12):1608–16.
38. Spagnolo R, Bonalumi M, Pace F, et al. Calcaneus fractures, results of the sinus tarsi approach: 4 years of experience. Eur J Orthop Surg Traumatol 2010;20: 37–42.
39. Acumed Calcaneal Plating System. Surgical Technique Guide. Effective 5/2011.
40. Tornier. the WAVE: Calcaneal fracture plate surgical technique guide. 2010.
41. Talarico LM, Vito GR, Zyryanov SY. Management of displaced intraarticular calcaneal fractures by using external ring fixation, minimally invasive open reduction, and early weightbearing. J Foot Ankle Surg 2004;43(1):43–50.
42. Kissel CG, Husain ZS, Cottom JM, et al. Early clinical and radiographic outcomes after treatment of displaced intra-articular calcaneal fractures using delta-frame external fixator construct. J Foot Ankle Surg 2011;50(2):135–40.
43. Gupta AK, Gluck GS, Parekh SG. Balloon reduction of displaced calcaneus fractures: surgical technique and case series. Foot Ankle Int 2011;32(2):205–10.
44. Stapleton JJ, Kolodenker G, Zgonis T. Internal and external fixation approaches to the surgical management of calcaneal fractures. Clin Podiatr Med Surg 2010;27(3):381–92.
45. Facaros Z, Ramanujam CL, Zgonis T. Primary subtalar joint arthrodesis with internal and external fixation for the repair of a diabetic comminuted calcaneal fracture. Clin Podiatr Med Surg 2011;28(1):203–9.
46. Longino D, Buckley RE. Bone graft in the operative treatment of displaced intra-articular calcaneal fractures: is it helpful? J Orthop Trauma 2001;15(4):280–6.
47. Pollard JD, Schuberth JM. Posterior bone block distraction arthrodesis of the subtalar joint: a review of 22 cases. J Foot Ankle Surg 2008;47(3):191–8.
48. Lee MS, Tallerico V. Distraction arthrodesis of the subtalar joint using allogeneic bone graft: a review of 15 cases. J Foot Ankle Surg 2010;49(4):369–74.
49. Beuerlein M, McKee M. Calcium sulfate: what is the evidence? J Orthop Trauma 2010;24(Suppl 3):S46–51.

50. Stannard JP, Robinson JT, Anderson ER, et al. Negative pressure wound therapy to treat hematomas and surgical incisions following high-energy trauma. J Trauma 2006;60(6):1301–6.
51. DeCarbo WT, Hyer CF. Negative-pressure wound therapy applied to high-risk surgical incisions. J Foot Ankle Surg 2010;49(3):299–300.
52. Wallace GF. Complications of heel surgery. Clin Podiatr Med Surg 2010;27(3): 393–406.
53. Heier KA, Infante AF, Walling AK, et al. Open fractures of the calcaneus: soft-tissue injury determines outcome. J Bone Joint Surg Am 2003;85(12):2276–82.
54. Schepers T, Kieboom BC, Bessems GH, et al. Subtalar versus triple arthrodesis after intra-articular calcaneal fractures. Strategies Trauma Limb Reconstr 2010; 5(2):97–103.

Tarsometatarsal/ Lisfranc Joint

Lawrence A. DiDomenico, DPM[a],*, Davi Cross, DPM[b]

KEYWORDS

- Lisfranc injury • Foot • Tarsus • Metatarsus

It has been projected that injuries to this region of the foot occur in approximately 1 in 55,000 people per year, encompassing 0.2% of all fractures; however, these numbers may be an underestimation.[1] It is the opinion and the experience of the authors that this injury occurs more commonly and the diagnosis is often unseen. It is common for foot and ankle specialist to evaluate patients with a Lisfranc injury days or weeks after a visit to the emergency room with an unrecognized injury. Subtle injuries can occur in the midfoot and are frequently missed by the initial evaluator as well the follow-up evaluations. A Lisfranc injury can be difficult to diagnose and may be unnoticed in patients who have experienced polytrauma (multiple injuries) or in patients who experience simple injuries such as a slip and or misstep. There are varying degrees of these injuries from a simple sprain to an unstable fracture/dislocation. Misdiagnosis and inappropriate treatment can lead to a painful long-term condition.

HISTORICAL REVIEW

During the Napoleonic era, the field surgeon Jacques Lisfranc encountered a patient who suffered from vascular compromise and secondary gangrene of the foot after a fall from a horse. Subsequently, Lisfranc performed an amputation at the level of the tarsometatarsal joints, and thereafter the eponym of Lisfranc joint has been applied to that area of the foot. Although Lisfranc did not describe a specific mechanism of injury or classification scheme for the injury within this region, a Lisfranc injury traditionally reflects a dislocation or fracture-type injury at the tarsometatarsal joints.

ANATOMY

Thorough comprehension of the osseous, capsular, and ligamentous structures encompassed within the tarsometatarsal joint complex is essential for appropriate diagnosis and treatment of disorders in that region.

The Lisfranc joint complex consists of the articulations of the intertarsal, intermetatarsal, and tarsometatarsal surfaces. This complex forms medial, central, and lateral

[a] 8175 Market Street, Youngstown, OH 44512, USA
[b] Heritage Valley Health System, 1000 Dutch Ridge Road, Beaver, PA, USA
* Corresponding author.
E-mail address: ld5353@aol.com

Clin Podiatr Med Surg 29 (2012) 221–242
doi:10.1016/j.cpm.2012.01.003
0891-8422/12/$ – see front matter © 2012 Elsevier Inc. All rights reserved.

columns, which together form an arch configuration through the midfoot (**Figs. 1 and 2**). Each of the columns is independent of the others, with unique synovial membranes.[2] The medial column is formed by the first metatarsal and medial cuneiform, the second column is formed by the second and third metatarsals and the intermediate and lateral cuneiforms, and the third column consists of the cuboid and its relationship with the fourth and fifth metatarsals.[2,3] Each of these columns possesses the following amount of sagittal plane motion: 3.5 mm, 0.6 mm, and 13 mm, respectively.[4] The base of the second metatarsal is recessed between the medial and lateral cuneiforms, and this placement is thought to provide much of the stability to the joint, by providing limitation in the amount of plantarflexion and dorsiflexion (**Fig. 3**).[5,6] In addition, the wedge-type shape of the base of the second metatarsal in conjunction with the shape of the other metatarsals is another component adding stability to the joint, because it gives stability in the frontal plane, which allows for enhanced function of the surrounding soft tissue structures.[7] In general, the osseous components of the joint are larger dorsally than plantarly.[2]

Fibrous membranes that are lined with synovium divide the complex into the 3 divisions, and are referred to as articular capsules.[2,8] These capsules insert at various bony articular surfaces within the complex.

The ligamentous structures throughout the Lisfranc joint have been found to have moderate variability in cadaver studies, and may or may not present as thickenings of the surrounding capsular linings.[2] Each structure is composed of longitudinal and oblique strands and, together, the ligaments are grouped into dorsal, interosseous, and plantar sections.[2] There are 6 to 8 ligaments in the dorsal group, and these flat structures conjoin the tarsal and metatarsal bones.[2] The interosseous ligament group contains 3 members, including the interosseous intercuneiform ligament, which has been found to provide significant stability to the joint. Another key stabilizing structure within this group and the overall joint complex is thought to be the Y-shaped ligament that connects the medial base of the second metatarsal to the lateral aspect of the medial cuneiform, and this is referred to as the Lisfranc ligament.[6] There is no intermetatarsal ligament between the base of the first and second metatarsals, and this may contribute to the propensity for dislocation-type injuries in this region.[9] There are traditionally at least 5 ligaments in the plantar ligament group, including the intertarsal and intermetatarsal components. These ligaments are stronger than their dorsal counterparts.[2]

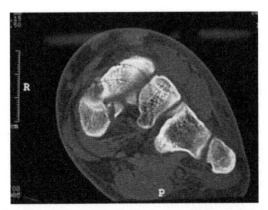

Fig. 1. A frontal plane view of a computed tomography (CT) scan showing an injury at the bases of the metatarsals.

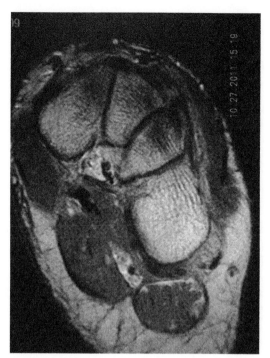

Fig. 2. A frontal plane view of a magnetic resonance imaging (MRI) scan of the medial, intermediate, and lateral cuneiforms and cuboid. Note the naturally occurring arch.

In an anatomic study of injured Lisfranc joints, it was determined that the mortise between the medial and lateral cuneiform bones was significantly shallower in people who had sustained injuries to the area, therefore suggesting that this anatomic difference may predispose certain individuals to damage to the joint.[6]

MECHANISM OF INJURY

In general, Lisfranc joint injury can be secondary to either direct or indirect trauma, and this mechanism determines the type of clinical presentation and the type of injury. Direct trauma involves a crushing-type injury, most likely to create a plantar dislocation of the metatarsals. Indirect trauma results from a rotational-type force across the joint with the eversion/pronation type being the most common.[7] Strong forces directed from lateral to medial often cause ligamentous rupture or fracture sites located at the second metatarsal base.[7] Eversion/pronation-type injuries can lead to medial dislocation of the first metatarsal, followed by dorsal and lateral dislocation of the lateral metatarsals.[7]

Most injuries at this joint result in displacement in a dorsal and lateral direction, because of the paucity and weakness of the surrounding dorsal and plantar ligamentous structures.[9] It has been found that, in injuries in which dislocation occurs, the dorsal tarsometatarsal ligaments are ruptured first, followed by the stronger plantar ligaments.[10] Stavlas and colleagues,[11] in their review of 11 articles examining outcomes in 257 patients with Lisfranc injuries, found that 57.5% of the patients had combined osseoligamentous injuries and 42.5% experienced purely ligamentous injury.

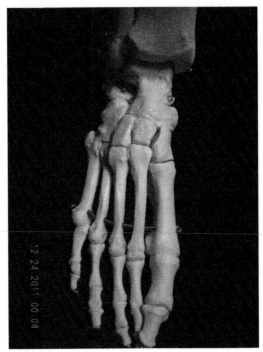

Fig. 3. The base of the second metatarsal is situated between the medial and lateral cuneiforms as well as the base of the first and third metatarsals.

Traditionally, the injury is more common in male patients who have suffered a high-energy indirect traumatic event, in which a rotational force has been applied to a plantarflexed foot.[3,4,9] Because of the mechanism of action related to this type of injury, they can be seen in athletic scenarios, but they are commonly seen in high-impact incidents such as motor vehicle and industrial accidents.[12,13]

INJURY CLASSIFICATIONS

A variety of classification schemes have been developed to describe injury to the Lisfranc joint complex. These systems typically describe anatomical radiographic variations of the anatomic injury pattern.

Quenu and Kuss[14] first described a straightforward classification detailing variations in tarsometatarsal injuries, which were classified as isolated, homolateral, and divergent, in 1909. Subsequent classifications described the injury primarily based on the mechanism of action, and some divided the injury based on the presence or absence of soft tissue spraining.[15] However, these did not address the method of treatment based on the appearance of the injury.

In 1982, Hardcastle and colleagues[13] modified the previously described Quenu and Kuss[14] model to provide a system that could dictate what treatment modality may be used based on the appearance of the injury. The classification was broken down into 3 groups, beginning with type A, which describes total uniplanar incongruity of the tarsometatarsal joint. Type B in this scheme entails partial displacement of either the first metatarsal or the remaining metatarsals, individually or together. Type C presents as any combination of displacement that always includes the first metatarsal in combination with any or all of the lesser metatarsals. This type typically also shows sagittal and frontal displacement.[13]

Myerson and colleagues[16] (1986) further developed the Hardcastle classification to describe the congruity of the joint as it related to the injury. This classification system is presently commonly used for this injury.

Postoperative functional outcomes after Lisfranc injury have been evaluated by several investigators.[5,7,17] Gaweda and colleagues[5] (2008), in their analysis of 19 patients, found that Hardcastle type B injuries showed the worst functional results, and they believed that this type of injury is most likely to be either misdiagnosed or undertreated.

DIAGNOSIS

A detailed history and physical examination is a key component to accurate and timely diagnosis of a Lisfranc injury. Injuries to the joint complex that result in subtle joint displacement are often difficult to diagnose clinically and radiographically. Many previously missed injuries have occurred in patients who dismissed their symptoms as resulting from a routine foot sprain, and later presented with lingering pain, swelling, or instability.[10]

Clinical examination should include evaluation of edema and ecchymosis, because typically there may be diffuse edema and plantar medial arch ecchymosis present in this type of injury (**Fig. 4**).[11,18] In addition, passive manipulation of the forefoot into pronation and supination allows for evaluation of stability of the joint complex.[18] Long-standing injuries that were previously misdiagnosed or undiagnosed show a variety of symptoms depending on the time span since, and severity of, the initial injury. These changes may include a flatfoot deformity stemming from the midfoot; pain with palpation over any of the metatarsocuneiform joints, specifically the second; or decreased arch height during heel rise.[10,15]

Diagnostic radiographic imaging should always be conducted for completeness of the examination. Weight-bearing radiographs taken in anteroposterior, lateral, and 30° oblique views can help to show frank diastasis as well as gross bony abnormalities (**Figs. 5–7**). If suspicion is high for soft tissue injury, radiographic stress views can be performed, either with or without anesthetic block (**Figs. 8** and **9**).[10] However,

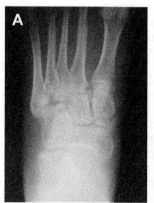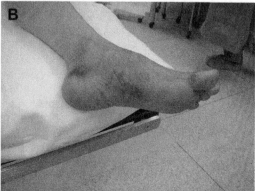

Fig. 4. (A) A fleck sign with gapping is noted at the intercuneiform and Lisfranc joint. (B) Clinically, there is residual edema and echymosis in the plantar medial arch, which is typically seen with Lisfranc injuries.

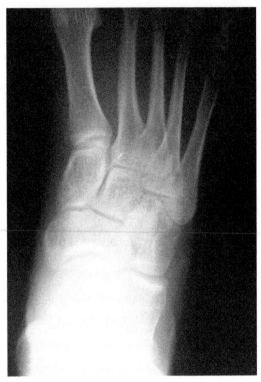

Fig. 5. An anterior-posterior and medial oblique radiograph with no abnormalities at the Lisfranc joint.

radiographic evaluation can be difficult, secondary to shadowing or overlapping that occurs between the metatarsal and tarsal bones.[19] Radiographic findings may include widening between the metatarsal bases, a fragmentary fracture at the medial base of the second metatarsal or lateral medial cuneiform, or displacement of the lesser meta-tarsals. Myerson[4] identified a fleck sign that can be seen at the medial base of the second metatarsal or lateral base of the first metatarsal as an avulsion fracture.

In injuries in which there is less than 2 mm of diastasis between the bases of meta-tarsals 1 and 2, magnetic resonance imaging (MRI) or computed tomography (CT) is the preferred imaging modality (**Figs. 10** and **11**).[20] Soft tissue structures can be thor-oughly evaluated by using MRI performed in various planes. In the oblique axial plane, the integrity of the Lisfranc ligament is visible, in addition to the overall alignment of the tarsal and metatarsal bones. The transverse arch of the foot can be evaluated in the frontal plane, and, in the sagittal plane, plantar and dorsal joint alignment as well as the tarsometatarsal ligaments can be viewed.[19] CT imaging has been described as the diagnostic tool of choice by some investigators, because it has been found to be more reliable than plain radiographs.[17]

Overall, timely diagnosis is thought to be the key for successful outcomes for patients with this injury. This factor has been examined in several studies, specifically on athletes, who typically desire to return to full activity. In his review of 15 patients treated for this injury, Saxena[21] found that a delay of diagnosis greater than 6 weeks decreased the chance of the patient having an excellent outcome. Posttraumatic

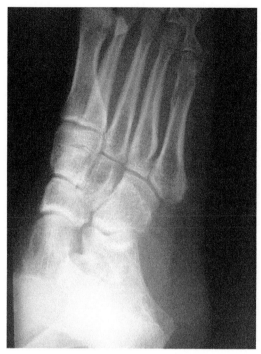

Fig. 6. An anterior-posterior and medial oblique radiograph with no abnormalities at the Lisfranc joint.

arthritis is common and is typically caused by articular surfaces damaged in the initial incident, poor anatomic reduction, or failure to recognize the injury.[4] The additional concern of neurovascular compromise associated with injuries to this area is paramount, and thus reinforces the principle of early diagnosis.[11,22] Hardcastle and colleagues[13] (1982) asserted that it was essential to perform open reduction of the injury if there seems to be vascular insufficiency to the foot after closed reduction has been performed.

TREATMENT

The aim of the treatment is to promptly create a stable, painless, plantigrade foot. This objective is achieved by anatomic reduction, alignment, and, if required, stable fixation. Delayed diagnosis of the injury, even when followed by appropriate correction of the deformity, typically results in poorer functional outcomes.[10,21] Proper anatomic reduction of the deformity has been shown to be a key component in the prevention of posttraumatic arthritis.[20,22]

Some investigators have proposed determining the treatment of choice based on whether there has been partial or complete ligamentous disruption.[23] In the group showing incomplete/partial ligamentous disruption, there are 3 stages of injury, each consisting of increasing amounts of diastasis within the joint. Also noted in this group is whether or not there is collapse of the medial arch. The treatment protocol for each of these types ranges from just symptomatic treatment to open reduction and internal fixation (ORIF). The other group, which entails complete disruption of the ligament, consists of 2 main subgroups: those without significant intra-articular

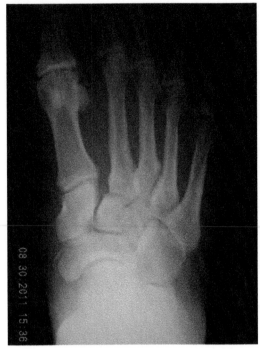

Fig. 7. An anterior-posterior view showing diastasis between the first and second metatarsal, a fleck sign, as well as the medial and intermediate cuneiform. Note the bone avulsion off the navicular.

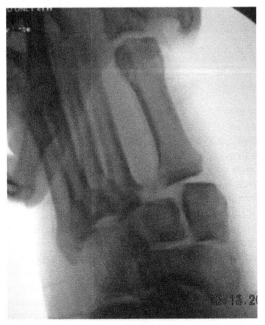

Fig. 8. Stress radiographs showing the instability at the tarsal metatarsal joints.

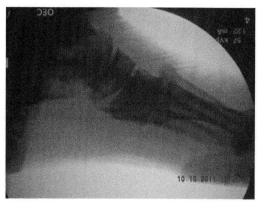

Fig. 9. A lateral radiograph showing instability in the sagittal plane.

fractures and those with comminuted intra-articular fractures. For these injuries, primary arthrodesis of the joint has been found to have more successful outcomes than those treated with ORIF.[23]

Conservative treatment of Lisfranc injuries is typically reserved for nondisplaced, stable injuries or fractures commonly seen with low-energy injuries. Some investigators have suggested that, for injuries more than 6 weeks old, without fracture, and without significant joint subluxation, conservative treatment is acceptable.[10] For this

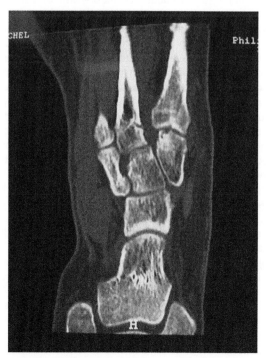

Fig. 10. CT scan showing disruption at the Lisfranc joint as well as a cuneiform fracture.

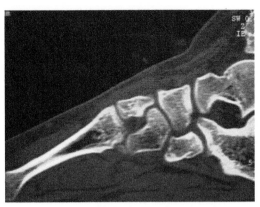

Fig. 11. CT scan showing disruption at the Lisfranc joint as well as a cuneiform fracture.

type of injury, a variety of modalities have been described, including below-knee immobilization and closed reduction with plaster casting; however, there is a risk of loss of reduction with these methods.[5,9,11,20] If closed reduction is to be attempted, some investigators have proposed using longitudinal traction followed by plantarflexion and supination of the forefoot, followed by dorsiflexion and pronation.[24] The authors suggest that patients who present with negative weight-bearing radiographs and a negative stress test can be managed well with a weight-bearing fracture boot.

If the Lisfranc complex shows a displacement of 2 mm or greater, anatomic reduction is necessary. If the fracture/dislocation is mobile and reducible, closed reduction should be attempted. However, postreduction radiographs are required to ensure adequate reduction and to ensure that no residual subluxation is noted. If closed reduction can be sustained, then a below-the-knee cast can be used as treatment alone.[25–28] Many investigators have suggested that closed reduction without fixation, either open or closed, does not maintain adequate reduction and often requires surgical stabilization.[29–32] Closed reduction should be attempted. If it does not maintain because of instability, reduction and fixation will be necessary.[13,33] In cases in which closed reduction cannot be maintained, open reduction and stable fixation is then mandatory and can be done via percutaneous pin and/or screw fixation (**Fig. 12**) (the authors routinely use screw fixation and do not believe k-wire fixation can provide an equally stable construct; **Fig. 13**). Placement of the percutaneous pin/screws depends on the type of injury. Fixation of the medial cuneiform to the second metatarsal base reconstitutes the Lisfranc ligament. If using k-wires, threaded k-wires provide better purchase than smooth k-wires, but are more difficult and more painful to remove.

Correction of deformity, maintaining anatomic alignment, in addition to the creation of a functional, stable plantigrade foot, are key components to surgical repair of this type of injury. Realignment typically is initiated at the medial column and then progressed laterally.[4] A plethora of internal and external fixation techniques for dislocation-type injuries has been described (**Figs. 14–25**). We prefer the use of a 4.0-mm solid cortical screw because the head is the same size as a 3.5-mm screw, the core diameter is 2.9 mm, and it is fully threaded and solid.

ORIF is the traditionally accepted treatment of displaced Lisfranc joint injuries. However, even with anatomic reduction and stable internal fixation, treatment of these injuries has not consistently provided excellent outcomes. Primary arthrodesis has

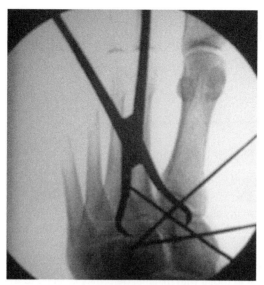

Fig. 12. An intraoperative view using a Weber clamp and k-wire fixation. The authors do not recommend k-wire fixation as a first-line option.

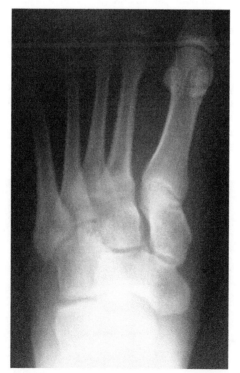

Fig. 13. Postoperative weight-bearing anterior-posterior radiograph showing a significant diastasis at the Lisfranc joint following k-wire fixation. This is the same patient as in **Fig. 12**, who had a poor result.

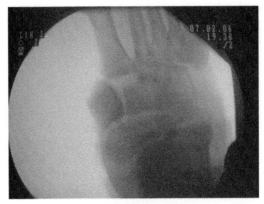

Fig. 14. A significant injury and displacement at the Lisfranc joint along with other involved midfoot joints.

also been shown to be a viable alternative for correction in scenarios in which there is severe dislocation or in those with minimal deformity isolated to the medial or middle columns.[4,15] Lateral column arthrodesis is typically unnecessary because those areas show few symptoms.[4] In the neuropathic patient, the authors suggest an arthrodesis of the lateral column when significant disorder is involved. In addition, diabetes mellitus with secondary Charcot neuropathic changes is responsible for most neuropathic fracture-dislocations. Joints that are unstable secondary to the neuropathic changes have a high rate of pseudoarthrosis resulting in the need to attempt a fusion.

It is common to need to remove hardware in patients who have received internal fixation, and this has been an issue in those receiving metallic as well as bioabsorbable hardware.[15]

Fractures with bony displacement are treated with external fixation or, more commonly, with traditional ORIF techniques. Open reduction provides a good means of achieving an anatomic reduction. Significant edema in the soft tissue envelop may impose a delay with open reduction of up to 14 to 21 days. The basic construct of open reduction consists of an interfragmentary compression screw (3.5-mm or

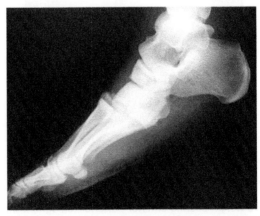

Fig. 15. A significant injury and displacement at the Lisfranc joint along with other involved midfoot joints.

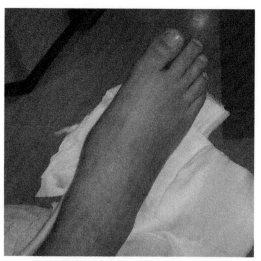

Fig. 16. Note the significant soft tissue injury secondary to the gross displacement of the bony structures; this can create a significant soft tissue injury.

4.0-mm fully threaded cortical screws) inserted into the second metatarsal base from the proximal superior-medial corner of the medial cuneiform. The initial compression screw is the key to the reduction and fixation of the injured complex, followed by multiple interfragmentary screws placed from the bases of the involved metatarsals to their respective cuneiform bones. If cuneiform instability is present, reduction and screw fixation between the cuneiforms can be inserted. In cases in which comminution of the cuneiform and metatarsal bases may be involved, this can be treated with bridge plating, allowing the surgeon to span the fracture and maintain anatomical alignment and length.

The standard incisional approach consist of 1 or 2 incisions. The most medial is slightly lateral and parallel to the first metatarsal shaft starting at the distal one-third

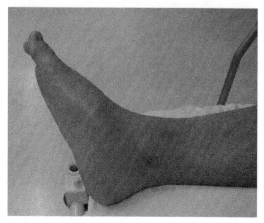

Fig. 17. Note the significant soft tissue injury secondary to the gross displacement of the bony structures; this can create a significant soft tissue injury.

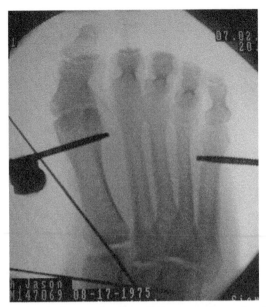

Fig. 18. Treatment consisted of protecting the soft tissue envelop and maintaining anatomic alignment with the use of an external fixator.

metatarsal and extending to the navicular. The authors recommend making the incision curvilinear over the first tarsal metatarsal. This technique can provide good exposure to the first, second, and third tarsal metatarsal joints while allowing the surgeon to retract the deep peroneal nerve and dorsalis pedis artery. When needed, the second incision should be over the fourth metatarsal shaft. The soft tissue island between the incisions needs to be adequate in size to prevent tissue necrosis. If only the medial tarsal metatarsal joints are involved, the authors make 1 large dorsal curvilinear incision starting at the dorsal lateral first metatarsal and extending to the

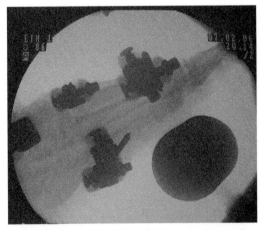

Fig. 19. Treatment consisted of protecting the soft tissue envelop and maintaining anatomic alignment with the use of an external fixator.

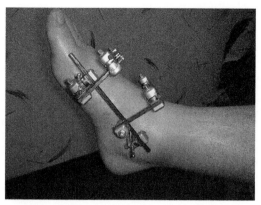

Fig. 20. Treatment consisted of protecting the soft tissue envelop and maintaining anatomic alignment with the use of an external fixator.

navicular-cuneiform joint. Care should be taken not to undermine/separate the tissues to prevent soft tissue damage. The incision is deepened to the extensor hallucis brevis tendon, which runs over the neurovascular bundle. The neurovascular bundle should be retracted to whichever side is easiest and allows the best exposure to provide excellent visualization to the base of the second metatarsal to the medial cuneiform as well as the second tarsal metatarsal joint. Identifiable bony fragments that are too small to be fixed are removed. Next, k-wires are used for temporary fixation until anatomic alignment is confirmed under fluoroscopy. A 3.5-mm or 4.0-mm fully threaded cortical screw with a lag technique should enter from the medial cuneiform

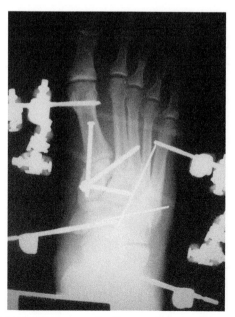

Fig. 21. A staged percutaneous screw fixation procedure was provided for additional stability, following a favorable response by the soft tissues.

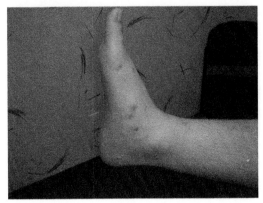

Fig. 22. After 10 weeks of fixation, the hardware was removed. Clinical and radiographic views show a well-aligned foot.

and be directed in an oblique fashion into the base of the second metatarsal. If instability is noted at the intercuneiforms (the more stabile proximal base), then an intercuneiform lag screw should be used from medial to lateral. If the lateral segments are disrupted, the second incision is used. The incision is deepened and attention should be directed to the third metatarsal tarsal base. Soft tissue or bony fragments that may be blocking the reduction are resected. A smooth k-wire is used for temporary fixation beginning at the third metatarsal base into the lateral cuneiform. Similar to ankle fractures, the Vassal principle applies to the Lisfranc complex. Once reduction of the

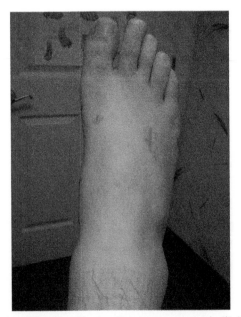

Fig. 23. After 10 weeks of fixation, the hardware was removed. Clinical and radiographic views show a well-aligned foot.

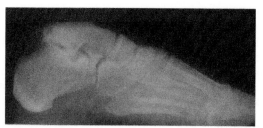

Fig. 24. After 10 weeks of fixation, the hardware was removed. Clinical and radiographic views show a well-aligned foot.

medial (dominant segment) tarsal metatarsal is successfully reduced, the remaining lesser tarsal metatarsal joints will find their natural anatomic location.

The postoperative course varies with the surgical protocol; the patient is placed in a dorsally slotted non–weight-bearing plaster cast for 2 weeks and instructed to keep

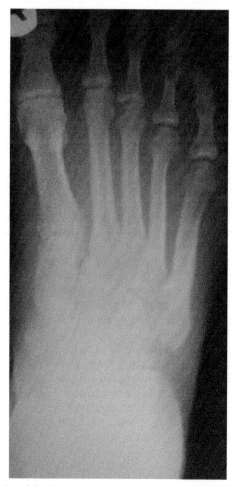

Fig. 25. After 10 weeks of fixation, the hardware was removed. Clinical and radiograph views show a well-aligned foot.

the extremity elevated. Provided there are no wound problems and the reduction and construct are stable, a below-the-knee fiberglass cast is applied for an additional 4 to 6 weeks. Full weight bearing in a fracture boot with physical therapy is then prescribed for 4 weeks. If percutaneous smooth or threaded k-wires have been used, they can be removed at approximately 8 weeks. If screws have been used, they can be removed at approximately 12 weeks. Full unprotected weight bearing is typically not permitted until hardware has been removed.[34]

ARTHRODESIS TECHNIQUE

In the patient who is non-neuropathic, typically the first, second, and/or third tarsal metatarsal joints are fused. A single curvilinear incision as described earlier is used. The neurovascular bundle is identified and retracted. The first, second, and/or third metatarsal cuneiform joints are exposed. The articular surfaces are debrided to bleeding bone while attempting to preserve as much of the natural integrity as possible, which minimizes the shortening bone voids. Osteotomes, mallets, picks, rongeurs, drills, and curettes are the instruments used for the debridement. A significant amount of time is spent on joint preparation because we believe that the success of an arthrodesis is in the joint preparation, alignment, and fixation construct. After adequate articular debridement, the reduction is performed using temporary k-wire fixation. The alignment is confirmed both clinically and with fluoroscopy. The stabilization is begun from proximal to distal with the cuneiforms. Once the cuneiforms are stabilized, the first tarsal metatarsal is temporarily fixated. It is important that the first metatarsal is in a neutral position and any varus/valgus position is corrected. In some scenarios, a temporary external fixator may need to be used for distraction. Next, the base of the second metatarsal is positioned appropriately into the native keystone position, followed by the third tarsal metatarsal. If the fourth and fifth metatarsal tarsal joints are involved, it has been the authors' experience that, once the first 3 tarsal metatarsal joints are positioned, the fourth and fifth metatarsal tarsal joints reduce anatomically. Fixation is achieved using a lag technique involving solid 3.5 or 4.0 cortical screws and/or plating techniques. A screw hole technique as described by Manoli and Hansen[35] allows for a difficult angulation and the first screw is inserted from the first metatarsal to the medial cuneiform, creating interfragmentary compression. The next screw is inserted from the stable superior proximal medial cuneiform, obliquely oriented into the second metatarsal base. Interfragmentary compression is also used at this stage. Additional screws can be inserted from the proximal metatarsal base into the cuneiform and from the base of the first metatarsal into the base of the second metatarsal (**Figs. 26** and **27**). All bone voids are then packed with autogenous or allogenic cancellous bone graft for a shear strain relief graft, as described by Perren.[36]

Postoperatively, the patient is placed in a dorsally slotted, non–weight-bearing plaster cast for 2 weeks and is instructed to keep the extremity elevated. Provided there are no wound problems and the reduction and construct are stable, a fiberglass below-the-knee cast is applied for an additional 4 to 6 weeks. Full weight bearing in a fracture boot with physical therapy is then prescribed for 4 weeks, followed by full weight bearing and regular activity. During the postoperative course, serial radiographs are taken until bony consolidation is noted.

COMPLICATIONS

Compartment syndrome is a serious condition that involves increased pressure in a muscle compartment. It can lead to muscle and nerve damage and problems with

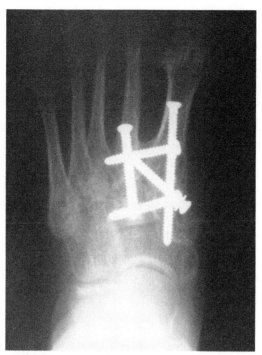

Fig. 26. An anterior-posterior radiograph showing a well-aligned midfoot following a primary arthrodesis after a Lisfranc injury.

blood flow. Heightened awareness assists the foot and ankle surgeon in avoiding the sequela of a missed compartment syndrome. Significant injuries to the midfoot can lead to prolonged ischemia, which may lead to irreversible destruction of myoneural tissue and subsequent fibrosis. Untreated compartment syndrome may lead to

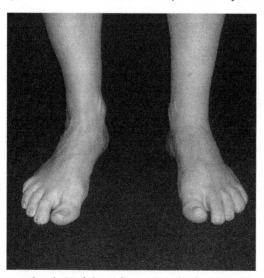

Fig. 27. After primary arthrodesis of the Lisfranc joint, the foot is stable, painless, and plantigrade, and the patient has minimal limitations.

a disabling outcome. The patient may experience chronic debilitating pain, and forefoot deformity such as residual claw toes. An intrinsic-minus deformity commonly
arises from interosseous and lumbrical muscle atrophy and subsequent fibrosis. In
addition, fibrosis of the short flexors secondary to the neural insult develops. Paresis
and anesthesia to the plantar foot may be permanent. Compartment syndrome of the
foot is a potentially disabling condition but is treatable if promptly recognized. Therefore, the foot and ankle surgeon must be highly suspicious, along with seeking objective evidence through pressure monitoring, to lessen the likelihood of this condition.

Additional injuries may consist of redislocation and circulatory compromise.[37,38] An
inevitable (and the most common) long-term complication is arthrosis.[31,38,39] However,
not all patients who develop radiographic degenerative changes are symptomatic.[16]
Arntz and colleagues[31] concluded that injuries to the articular surface and anatomic
reduction were the most important determinants in the development of posttraumatic
arthritis. Injuries to the deep peroneal nerve or dorsal pedis artery may occur. In cases
in which k-wires have been used, loss of fixation and/or reduction is possible. Other
complications consist of cellulitis/wound infection, contractures, complex regional
pain syndrome, posttraumatic arthritis, hardware failure, broken screws, deep venous
thrombosis, pulmonary embolism, incomplete reduction, redislocation, chronic pain,
posttraumatic arthritis/deformity (planovalgus), difficulty wearing shoes, chronic pain,
and malalignment.

DISCUSSION

Accurate early diagnosis with adequate reduction and maintenance of anatomic alignment of the dislocation or fracture within the Lisfranc joint complex have been found to
be the key to successful outcomes regarding this injury. Because of the anatomic variations, the thin soft tissue envelop, and the abundance of ligamentous and capsular
structures in the region, repair of these injuries can be a challenge. The classification
systems used to describe these injuries aid in describing the mechanism of injury or
displacement type present, which may aid in determining what treatment modality
can provide the best outcome.

REFERENCES

1. Rosenberg GA, Patterson BM. Tarsometatarsal (Lisfranc's) fracture-dislocation.
   Am J Orthop (Belle Mead NJ) 1995;(Suppl):7–16.
2. DePalma L, Santucci A, Sabetta S, et al. Anatomy of the Lisfranc joint complex.
   Foot Ankle Int 1997;18(6):356–64.
3. Scolaro J, Ahn J, Mehta S. Lisfranc fracture dislocations. Clin Orthop Relat Res
   2011;469:2078–80.
4. Myerson MS. The diagnosis and treatment of injury to the tarsometatarsal joint
   complex. J Bone Joint Surg Br 1999;81(5):756–63.
5. Gaweda K, Tarczynska M, Modrzewski K, et al. An analysis of pathomorphic
   forms and diagnostic difficulties in tarso-metatarsal joint injuries. Int Orthop
   2008;32:705–10.
6. Peicha G, Labovitz J, Seibert FJ, et al. The anatomy of the joint as a risk factor for
   Lisfranc dislocation and fracture-dislocation. An anatomical and radiological
   case control study. J Bone Joint Surg Br 2002;84(7):981–5.
7. Van der Werf GJ, Tonio AJ. Tarsometatarsal fracture-dislocation. Acta Orthop
   Scand 1984;55:647–51.
8. Makwana NK. Tarsometatarsal injuries-Lisfranc injuries. Curr Orthop 2005;19:
   108–18.

9. Philbin T, Rosenberg G, Sferra JJ. Complications of missed or untreated Lisfranc injuries. Foot Ankle Clin 2003;8:61–71.
10. Aronow MS. Treatment of the missed Lisfranc injury. Foot Ankle Clin 2006;11: 127–42.
11. Stavlas P, Roberts CS, Xypnitos FN, et al. The role of reduction and internal fixation of Lisfranc fracture-dislocations: a systematic review of the literature. Int Orthop 2010;34:1083–91.
12. DeOrio M, Erickson M, Usuelli FG, et al. Lisfranc injuries in sport. Foot Ankle Clin 2009;14:169–86.
13. Hardcastle PH, Reschauer R, Kutscha-Lissberg E, et al. Injuries to the tarsometatarsal joint. J Bone Joint Surg Br 1982;64(3):349–56.
14. Quenu E, Kuss G. Etude sur les luxations du metatarse. Rev Chir Paris 1909;39: 281 [in French].
15. Chaney M. The Lisfranc joint. Clin Podiatr Med Surg 2010;27:547–60.
16. Myerson MS, Fisher RT, Burgess AR, et al. Fracture dislocations of the tarsometatarsal joints: end results correlated with pathology and treatment. Foot Ankle 1986;6(5):225–42.
17. Meirsch D, Wild M, Jungbluth P, et al. A transcuneiform fracture-dislocation of the midfoot. Foot (Edinb) 2011;21:45–7.
18. Rhim B, Hunt JC. Lisfranc injury and Jones fracture in sports. Clin Podiatr Med Surg 2011;28:69–86.
19. Preidler KW, Brossmann J, Daenen B, et al. MR imaging of the tarsometatarsal joint: analysis of injury in 11 patients. Am J Roentgenol 1996;167:1217–22.
20. Zgonis T, Roukis TS, Polyzois VD. Lisfranc fracture-dislocations: current treatment and new surgical approaches. Clin Podiatr Med Surg 2006;23:303–22.
21. Saxena A. Bioabsorbable screws for reduction of Lisfranc's diastasis in athletes. J Foot Ankle Surg 2005;44(6):445–9.
22. Wilppula E. Tarsometatarsal fracture-dislocation: late results in 26 patients. Acta Orthop Scand 1973;44:335–45.
23. Coetzee JC. Making sense of Lisfranc injuries. Foot Ankle Clin 2008;13:695–704.
24. Mulier T, Reynders P, Sioen W, et al. The treatment of Lisfranc injuries. Acta Orthop Belg 1997;63(2):82–90.
25. Lisfranc J. Nouvelle methode operatoire pour l'amputation partielle du pied par son articulation tarso-metatarsienne. Paris: L'imprimerie de Feuguery; 1815 [in French].
26. Foster SC, Foster RR. Lisfranc's tarsometatarsal fracture-dislocation. Radiology 1976;120:79–83.
27. Trevino SG, Kodros S. Controversies in tarsometatarsal injuries. Orthop Clin North Am 1995;26:229–38.
28. Gissane W. A dangerous type of fracture of the foot. J Bone Joint Surg Br 1951; 33:535.
29. Meyer SA, Callaghan JJ, Albright JP, et al. Midfoot sprains in collegiate football players. Am J Sports Med 1994;22:392–401.
30. Myerson M. The diagnosis and treatment of injuries of the Lisfranc joint complex. Orthop Clin North Am 1989;20:655–64.
31. Arntz CT, Veith RG, Hansen ST. Fractures and fracture-dislocations of the tarsometatarsal joint. J Bone Joint Surg 1988;70:173.
32. Goosens M, De Stoop N. Lisfranc's fracture-dislocations: etiology, radiology, and results of treatment. Clin Orthop 1983;176:154–62.
33. Granberry WM, Liscomb PR. Dislocations of the tarsometatarsal joints. Surg Gynecol Obstet 1962;114:467–9.

34. Harwood MI, Raikin SM. A Lisfranc fracture-dislocation in a football player. J Am Board Fam Pract 2003;16:69–72.
35. Manoli A II, Hansen ST Jr. Screw hole preparation in foot surgery. Foot Ankle Int 1990;11:105–6.
36. Perren SM. Physical and biological aspects of fracture healing with special reference to internal fixation. Clin Orthop Relat Res 1979;138:175–96.
37. Banks AS, Downey MS, Martin DE, et al. McGlammry's comprehensive textbook of foot and ankle surgery. 3rd edition. Philadelphia: Lippincott Williams & Wilkins; 2011. p. 1742.
38. Bassett FH. Dislocations of the tarsometatarsal joints. South Med J 1964;57: 1294–302.
39. Thompson MC, Mormino MA. Injury to the tarsometatarsal joint complex. J Am Acad Orthop Surg 2003;11:260–7.

Pilon Fractures

Denise M. Mandi, DPM[a],*, Ron P. Belin, DPM[a], Justin Banks[b],
Brandon Barrett[b]

KEYWORDS

- Pilon fractures • Tibial/fibular fractures • Distal tibial fractures
- Plafond fractures

Pilon fractures are the ugly cousin of the ankle fracture. Unstable, often open, technically challenging and wrought with less-than-ideal outcomes, they are the bane of even the most experienced of surgeons. These devastating injuries are rare, comprising only 3% to 10% of all tibial fractures and 1% of all lower extremity fractures.[1]

Pilon fractures occur in the distal tibia as a result of low-energy twisting or high-energy axial forces caused by falls from a height or motor vehicle accidents, producing an array of tibial articular and metaphyseal injuries, with or without fracture of the fibula.[2–9] These fractures usually involve a significant portion of the weight-bearing articular surface, and, because of the extent of ankle joint involvement, these fractures can be problematic to treat and difficult to fixate.[10] The term pilon was first coined in 1911 by French radiologist Etienne Destot, and is the French word for pestle.[1] In 1950, Bonnin named these injuries plafond fractures, focusing on the articular involvement.[11]

A pilon fracture occurs when the talus is driven up into the distal tibial articular surface, or plafond. Anatomic differences between the tibial plafond and talar trochlea determine the result of a collision between the 2 bones. The smaller, relatively flat surface of the plafond compared with the larger, convex dome shape of the talus, and fewer internal trabeculae to reinforce the plafond compared with the talar dome, cause the tibial plafond to be most likely to fracture when the 2 bones collide.[12] This fracture results in comminution of the metaphysis and impaction of the articular surface.[13] The varying degrees of impaction that the supramalleolar metaphysis shows distinguishes the pilon fracture from the simpler trimalleolar ankle fracture. The high-energy impact causes comminution, articular surface destruction, and considerable soft tissue damage, which often contribute to unsatisfactory outcomes **(Figs. 1–4)**.[10,14]

In the early 1960s, the Association for Osteosynthesis/Orthopaedic Trauma (AO/OTA) developed guidelines for treating distal tibial articular surface fractures, which led to open reduction and anatomic rigid internal fixation of these fractures. In 1969,

[a] Section of Foot & Ankle Surgery, Department of Surgery, Broadlawns Medical Center, 1801 Hickman Road, Des Moines, IA 50314, USA
[b] Des Moines University, 3200 Grand Avenue, Des Moines, IA 50312, USA
* Corresponding author.
E-mail address: dmandi@broadlawns.org

Clin Podiatr Med Surg 29 (2012) 243–278
doi:10.1016/j.cpm.2012.01.001   **podiatric.theclinics.com**
0891-8422/12/$ – see front matter © 2012 Elsevier Inc. All rights reserved.

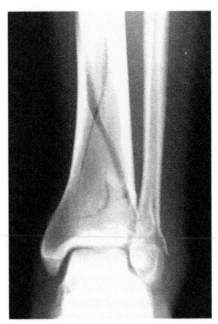

Fig. 1. Pilon fracture from low-energy twisting injury, preoperative anteroposterior view.

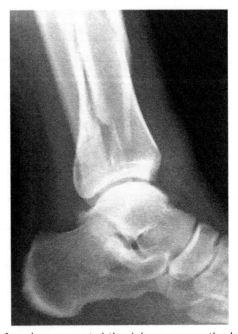

Fig. 2. Pilon fracture from low-energy twisting injury, preoperative lateral view.

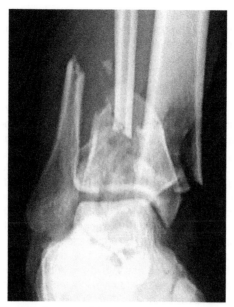

Fig. 3. Pilon fracture from high-energy injury, preoperative anteroposteior view.

Ruedi and Allgower reported promising results when treating patients with pilon fractures using these recommended guidelines.[6]

Controversy still exists about how to best treat these injuries, but most clinicians advocate surgical intervention unless contraindicated, with some combination of open reduction with internal fixation (ORIF) or external fixation.[15,16] Treatment goals

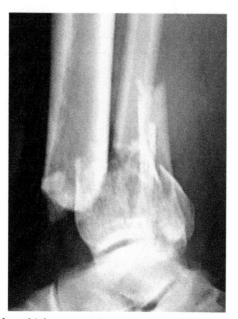

Fig. 4. Pilon fracture from high-energy injury, preoperative lateral view.

include anatomic reduction of the articular surface, reestablishment of length, preservation of axial alignment, correction of rotation, and early motion of the ankle.[16,17] Even when these goals are achieved, there is no guarantee that results will be acceptable.[18]

CLASSIFICATION

Destot divided pilon fractures into 4 main subgroups: posterior marginal (isolated posterior malleolar fractures), anterior marginal (isolated anterior tibial lip fractures), explosion, and supra-articular.[12] This was neither a descriptive nor comprehensive classification system, and did nothing to guide treatment or predict outcomes.

The AO classification scheme was designed to allow for detailed description of the various types of pilon fractures. This classification system is useful in research, but is the most complex of the classification schemes.[16] Pilon fractures in the AO scheme have been divided based on the degree of involvement of the articular surface. Type A fractures are extracapsular, type B fractures are partially articular, and type C fractures are completely articular. To further classify these injuries, types A, B, and C fractures can be subdivided into stages 1, 2, or 3. Stage 1 lacks comminution of the metaphysis or the epiphysis. Stage 2 involves impaction or comminution of the metaphysis but not the epiphysis. Stage 3 presents with comminution and impaction of both the metaphysis and the epiphysis **(Fig. 5)**.[19,20]

In 1969, Ruedi and Allgower[6] studied 84 pilon fractures and developed a classification system based on the degree of displacement, comminution, and impaction of the fracture fragments. They divided the pilon fractures into 3 subgroups: type I fractures

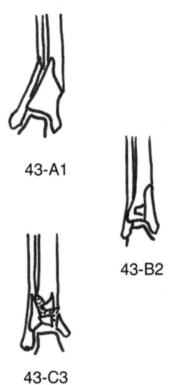

43-A1

43-B2

43-C3

Fig. 5. AO classification scheme for pilon fractures.

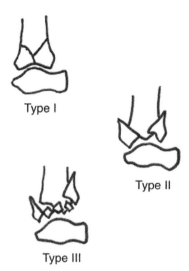

Type I

Type II

Type III

Fig. 6. Ruedi-Allgower classification scheme for pilon fractures.

show distal tibial fracture without comminution or displacement, type II fractures show dislocation at the ankle, but lack comminution or impaction, and type III fractures present with impacted and severely comminuted fragments of the distal tibia. They further discovered that the most severe pilon fractures were the most common, with 47% type III, 28% type II and 25% type I, respectively.[10] Theirs is the most widely used classification system currently available (**Fig. 6**).

Of additional interest, because 10% to 30% of all pilon fractures are open,[21] is the Tscherne soft tissue injury classification system (**Table 1**).[22]

OVERVIEW

The consensus description of a pilon fracture consists of a distal tibial fracture, often intra-articular and comminuted, that sometimes involves a fibular fracture; can be caused by twisting, but most commonly by high-energy trauma or a fall from a height. Clearly, this is a fracture pattern that is difficult to nail down, and even more difficult to treat successfully. Crist and colleagues describe it well in their article on pilon fractures, "Outcomes are unpredictable because of fracture characteristics (ie, impaction, comminution, articular cartilage damage, residual joint incongruity), the risk of soft-tissue complications, and preinjury patient factors."[23] Certain common findings and overriding principles need to be taken into account in the surgical planning before repair of these perplexing injuries.

Table 1		
The Tscherne soft tissue injury classification system		
Grade	**Description**	**Fracture Pattern**
C 0	Little or no soft tissue injury	Mild
C I	Superficial abrasion	Mild to moderate
C II	Deep abrasion or local muscle contusion	Moderately severe
C III	Extensive skin contusion, crushing or muscle injury	Severe injury

In their comprehensive study of anatomy of pilon fractures of the distal tibia, Topliss and colleagues[24] stated, "The pilon fracture has a number of components, namely, the proximal extension, the fracture of the fibula with its relationships and, probably the most important, the articular fracture. Although all parts are associated, the problems which they present are different and it is logical therefore to consider them separately." These investigators believed that there are 2 distinct fracture families, the sagittal and the coronal, and that they are determined by "the degree of transfer of energy at the time of injury, the direction of the force and to a less degree, the age of the patient."

In his review, Sirkin[18] describes "three articular parts typically found in pilon fractures–the posterolateral fragment or Volkmann fragment, the medial malleolus fragment, and the anterolateral or Chaput fragment. In addition, there are three typical areas of comminution or impaction." Sirkin went on to describe lateral comminution between the anterolateral and posterolateral fragment near the fibula; central comminution; and medial shoulder comminution near the medial malleolus.[18]

Axial compression and rotation, acting independently or together, influence the fracture pattern. Axial load, usually as a result of high-energy trauma, causes the talar dome to affect the distal tibia, yielding metaphyseal comminution, articular fracture, and severe soft tissue disruption. Rotational forces, associated with low-energy trauma, cause plafond fractures with spiral extension into the tibial shaft.[10]

Whether the fibula is fractured along with the tibia is a matter of injury mechanics. Varus compression causes an oblique medial malleolar fracture, with the tibial shaft left in varus. The fibula remains intact, as well as the lateral and posterior tibial cortex. Often, when the fibula remains intact, the talofibular ligaments may be torn. The deltoid ligaments are nearly always intact, permitting reduction of some of the tibial fracture fragments by ligamentotaxis.[17] In fractures in which the fibula remains intact, it helps to maintain the length of the limb.[12]

Fibular fracture in pilon fracture is associated with severe tibial metaphyseal fracture and cortical insult.[25] Fracture of the fibula occurs in 75% to 85% of all pilon fractures.[6,26,27] Valgus shear fractures the fibula, leaving the tibial shaft in a valgus or neutral position.[3] This mechanism is often associated with open fracture, because of the valgus-induced tension placed on the thin skin overlying the medial malleolus.[25] In their anatomic study, Topliss and colleagues[24] found that there is occasionally ligamentous diastasis between the tibia and fibula, but more often, in 44% of their patients, there was "disruption of the normal tibiofibular relationship through bone," namely, a Chaput-type avulsion fracture of the anterolateral tibial fragment. These investigators noted that failure to recognize and correct this fracture pattern, or functional diastasis, could result in a widened mortise and residual ankle joint instability. Topliss and colleagues[24] also noted that insufficient restoration of the normal relationship between the talus and fibula in these fractures could likewise alter the normal biomechanics and function of the ankle joint. Similar to the relationship between the fibula and talus in ankle fractures described by Yablon and colleagues, "the talus faithfully followed…the lateral malleolus,"[28] in this instance, reduction of talofibular malposition helps to restore the lateral tibial fracture fragment, because it follows the fibula as a result of their attachment at the anterior inferior tibiofibular ligament (AITFL).

In 1969, Ruedi and Allgower[6] compared ORIF with conservative treatment of pilon fractures. Their results showed improved outcomes in those patients who underwent ORIF. Although ORIF allows direct visualization and optimal reduction of the articular surface and metaphyseal fragments, the potential for soft tissue complications is higher.[8,29–31] The mechanism of injury in most of Ruedi and Allgower's patients was a twisting fall while skiing, which typically involves less severe soft tissue injuries.[3] Extrapolation of Ruedi and Allgower's principles to the more common high-energy pilon fractures did not give comparable results.[4,13,32–35] Those fractures that were a result of high-energy injury showed a marked increase in complications, such as skin slough, dehiscence, infection, nonunion and malunion, and posttraumatic arthritis.[29,34] This information changed the landscape for pilon fracture management. The current trend is toward a combination of external fixation with or without limited internal fixation as the first-line treatment of complicated, high-energy pilon fractures.[35–37] Specifically, displaced pilon fractures with considerable comminution and soft tissue injury are currently treated with immediate ORIF of the distal fibular fracture and delayed ORIF of the tibial plafond by various approaches requiring external fixation.[31,38–41]

Crist and colleagues[23] asserted that "The soft-tissue injury associated with pilon fractures generally reflects the amount of energy absorbed at the time of injury and directly reflects the mechanism of injury … limiting and/or delaying surgical trauma is often valuable in protecting the soft-tissue envelope." In pilon fractures, therefore, it is the condition of the soft tissue that dictates the timing and often the method of repair, and careful operative planning is more important in the pilon fracture than perhaps any other lower extremity surgery.[31,38,42]

OPERATIVE PLANNING

When you approach a patient in your practice with a pilon fracture, look at the big picture first before getting caught up in the details. One-third to one-half of pilon fractures have other associated injuries or fractures. The literature reports that from 10% to 50% of pilon fractures are open fractures that can cause significant soft tissue damage.[2,25,32,43] Because these fractures are usually associated with high-energy trauma or a fall from a height, they represent major trauma and should be treated as such, necessitating lumbar and cervical spine films to rule out vertebral fracture, urinalysis to rule out bladder or kidney damage, and examination of the contralateral limb for fracture, and so forth. Fracture of the contralateral calcaneus and tibial shaft are most commonly found.[25] Fracture of the tibial plateau, talus (rare), proximal fibula, femur, pelvis, acetabulum, and lumbar spine are occasionally seen.[2,3,25,26,32,44–46]

Of particular interest in closed pilon fractures is the possibility of compartment syndrome. The early signs of severe pain, first webspace loss of sensorium, and weakness of toe dorsiflexion should raise concern before pulselessness or palor is noted.[10] Pain on passive dorsiflexion of the toes, weakness in toe flexion, and plantar hyperesthesia are signs of deep posterior compartment syndrome, and should be monitored closely.[25] The fact that a fracture is closed is no guarantee that it will remain a closed fracture. Immediate fracture reduction is often necessary to prevent skin compromise, conversion to open fracture, and associated infection and incision placement concerns.[23]

Historically, pilon distal tibial fractures were treated conservatively: "Skeletal traction through the os calcis was the standard treatment and post-traumatic osteoarthritis and stiffness the rule."[47] More than 40 years ago, Ruedi and Allgower[6] established the guidelines that directed treatment of pilon fractures, namely (1) reduction and stabilization of associated fibular fracture to restore lateral length, (2) anatomic restoration of the articular surface of the tibia, (3) bone grafting of metaphyseal defects, and (4) buttress plating of medial tibia to prevent varus deformation and allow early ankle joint motion.

Clinical research from the mid-1980s to the early 2000s on cases using immediate ORIF showed wound complication rates of up to 100%.[31,35,38,48–50] The condition of the soft tissues determines the choice of procedure, based on the individual situation.[17,29,51] Sommer[17] stated, "In cases with critical soft tissue injuries as well as in open fractures, it may be advisable to proceed in sequential steps."[29,51–54]

Surgeons have moved away from immediate ORIF of pilon fractures with soft tissue damage toward early limited stabilizing fixation, external fixation, and delayed definitive ORIF, but the treatment of choice in these complex cases remains controversial. Leonard and colleagues[32,55–58] affirmed, "What has been made definitively clear in the literature is that minimizing soft tissue damage is essential to prevent potentially severe complications such as wound breakdown, osteomyelitis, infected nonunions, and amputations." Many investigators have reported reduced soft tissue complications with the use of minimally invasive techniques, including initial stabilization of the fracture by external fixation and delay of miniopen or minimally invasive plate osteosynthesis (MIPO) until soft tissue recovery, and using percutaneous screws and tunneled plating.[39,59] Wyrsch and colleagues[35] and Vidyadhara and Rao,[60] in a prospective randomized trial of ORIF versus external fixation of pilon fractures, found that external fixation yielded clinical outcomes similar to those found with ORIF, but with significantly fewer complications. In 2000, Watson and colleagues[49] stated, "Interestingly, it was felt that the worse the initial soft tissue injury was, the poorer the overall function tended to be, regardless of the initial fracture pattern."

In support of Ilizarov external ring fixation for pilon fractures, Vidyadhara and Rao[60] proposed that "closed reduction, although less anatomic, is better than anatomic open reduction in high-energy tibial pilon fractures with articular disorganization...any treatment method should try first and foremost to limit soft tissue damage and avoid additional complications." Other investigators disagree, citing that although external fixation with or without limited internal fixation reduces the rate of soft tissue-related complications, they are limited in their ability to provide anatomic restoration of the articular surface or the mechanical axes, or to provide adequate stabilization.[38,48,49] However, Crist and colleagues[23] state that, "Although anatomic articular reduction is the historical standard and is associated with [a decrease in] the development of radiographic arthritis, it may not be critical to functional outcome." Clearly, there are arguments that can be backed up by research findings to support nearly any method of treatment of pilon fractures (save conservative treatment, which is reserved for the patients who are poor surgical risks), from immediate ORIF, to MIPO, to external fixation, hybrid fixation and any combination of these.[18,23,31,38,42,61]

Any surgeon with lower extremity trauma experience has probably fixed pilon fractures in a variety of fashions, trying to find the combination of techniques that optimizes results. At Broadlawns, we have evolved from immediate ORIF, to delayed ORIF, to combined limited ORIF and external fixation with delayed definitive ORIF (if needed). We have noted little difference in the outcomes, regardless of the technique chosen. Currently, we use a staged approach to pilon fractures, with immediate closed reduction (if necessary), immobilization in a Jones compression dressing and posterior splint, initial gross reduction of the tibial fracture by external fixation and ORIF of the fibula after 7 to 10 days of soft tissue recovery, and eventual definitive ORIF of the tibia (if necessary). Initial gross reduction by ORIF of the fibula and placement of an external fixator contributes to stability and restores limb length, and ligamentotaxis helps to preliminarily reduce the tibial fracture fragments. It is crucial to reestablish fibular length, rotation, and alignment during ORIF, not only to maintain ankle joint alignment, but to aid in the anatomic reduction of the tibial fracture.[62]

Delay of definitive reconstruction until soft tissue swelling has decreased (at least 10 days) was shown by multiple investigators to be beneficial. Wagner and Jakob[63] showed that the occurrence of soft tissue-related problems in tibial plateau fractures was highest when surgery was performed within 7 days of the injury. Wyrsch and colleagues[35] showed that surgery on distal tibial fractures within 3 to 5 days of injury led to the following complications: infection, 28%; wound issues, 33%; and

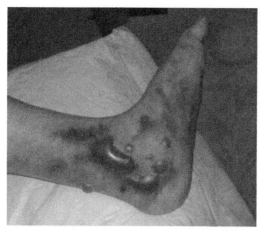

Fig. 7. Fracture blisters.

amputation, 16%. After pilon fracture, swelling caused by inflammation peaks at 12 to 24 hours after injury. Intradermal edema continues and peaks at 12 to 36 hours after injury. Fracture blisters occur in approximately one-third of patients. Blisters with clear fluid (intradermal blisters) are less alarming than blisters with hemorrhagic fluid (subdermal blisters), because the latter is a sign of more significant soft tissue damage, which should caution the surgeon against early ORIF (**Fig. 7**).[64]

Although pilon fractures are routinely diagnosed by clinical findings correlated with radiography of the injured and uninjured limbs, computed tomography (CT) is all but required in the planning of surgical intervention. Some investigators recommend

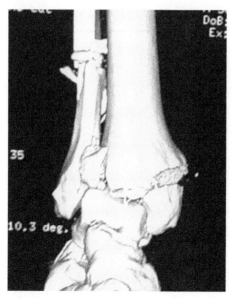

Fig. 8. Three-dimensional CT reconstruction of pilon fracture, anteroposterior view.

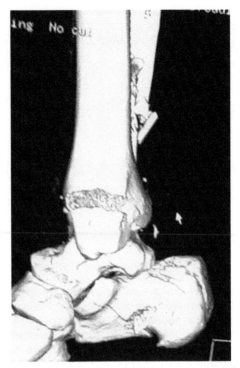

Fig. 9. Three-dimensional CT reconstruction of pilon fracture, medial view.

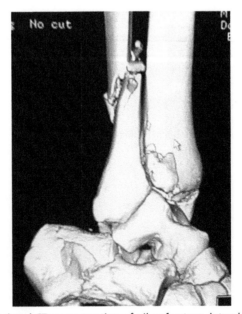

Fig. 10. Three-dimensional CT reconstruction of pilon fracture, lateral view.

immediate CT, whereas others recommend CT only after initial ORIF of the fibula (if needed) and provisional external fixation.[23,62] Topliss and colleagues[24] and Tornetta and Gorup[65] found that CT added information in 82% of patients and changed the proposed surgical plan in 64% of patients (**Figs. 8–10**).

Preoperative templating is more useful in pilon fracture surgical planning than in any other lower extremity surgery. After CT scan, fracture lines and fragment location should be templated and the approach to putting this complex puzzle together mapped out. Reconstruction of the articular surface should be performed first, because step-off in the joint surface is unacceptable, yet some malalignment of the tibia shaft can be tolerated, so shaft reduction is secondary.[16] Generally, the reassembly of the articular surface proceeds from posterior to anterior and from lateral to medial, with the medial malleolar fracture fragment acting as the final piece to complete the puzzle.[16]

METHODS
Closed Reduction

Because most pilon fractures are intra-articular, closed reduction of pilon fractures provides good results in only 43% to 50% of cases.[66] Most surgeons agree that anatomic reduction of the joint surface and early mobilization of the joint are the treatment goals in pilon fractures, which limits the usefulness of closed reduction to those patients who are poor surgical candidates, or as a component of a staged surgical procedure.[2,3,5,7,10,25,26,33,37,44,57,58,66–81]

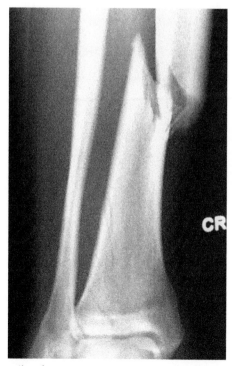

Fig. 11. Twisting injury pilon fracture, preoperative anteroposterior view.

Skeletal Traction

Skeletal traction has been used adjunctively with closed reduction, and remains a viable alternative treatment of nondisplaced, low-energy pilon fractures or in patients who are not surgical candidates because of debilitation or comorbidities.[2,7,9,26,44,46,82–85] In the face of severe comminution and impaction of the articular surface, traction fails, because there are no soft tissues attached to the articular fragments to aid in reduction.[10] Sanders and Stewart[16] go so far as to say, "It must be emphasized that calcaneal skeletal traction, even with the leg on a Bohler-Braun frame, has essentially no place in the treatment of these fractures."

Open Treatment

Application of the principles of AO/ASIF fracture fixation in the treatment of pilon fractures can lead to significant soft tissue complications if the fragile, damaged soft tissue envelope surrounding the fracture is not considered.

Because 10% to 50% of pilon fractures are open fractures, and the risk of compartment syndrome is high with these fractures, some type of stabilizing treatment may be required emergently. Franklin and colleagues[86] recommended a treatment protocol for open fractures including immediate irrigation and debridement of wounds, rigid fixation of all fractures, 48 hours of prophylactic antibiotics, and delayed primary skin closure after 5 days. The senior author (DMM) follows Gustilo and Anderson's

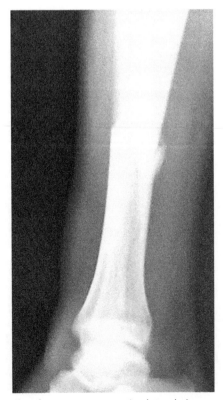

Fig. 12. Twisting injury pilon fracture, preoperative lateral view.

guidelines[87]: tetanus prophylaxis, empiric antibiotic therapy, and surgical irrigation and debridement to convert a contaminated wound to a clean wound.

Consideration of the state of the soft tissue envelope cannot be stressed enough in the treatment of pilon fractures: timing is everything. Initial edema is the result of short-ening of the limb and fracture hematoma formation.[26] Eight to twelve hours after injury, intradermal edema is present, which increases the risk of postoperative complica-tions; control of intradermal edema is key in successful wound healing.[10,26,46,88] The application of a Jones compression dressing and posterior splint coupled with ice and elevation for 7 to 10 days is the regimen that we follow. Delaying definitive treat-ment of pilon fractures until this edema is reduced is necessary to minimize the risk of postoperative complications, yet delaying past 4 weeks can make anatomic reduction of the fracture difficult at best: fracture hematoma begins to organize, osteoclastic activity rounds off the sharp fracture edges, and muscle contraction makes reduction almost impossible.[10,25,77,89]

Incision placement for open reduction must first consider existing lacerations, if the fracture is open, and next must respect underlying structures and blood supply. If multiple incisions are proposed (as is common), at least 7 to 8 cm of intact skin must be left as a bridge between the 2 incisions.[2,7,26,45,77,88,90,91] In their recent article proposing a single-incision lateral approach to pilon fractures, Femino and Vasee-non[41] state, "Knowledge of the angiosomes and vascular anatomy of skin over the ankle would make the length of parallel incisions and the skin bridge between the edges of the bipedicle flap created by parallel incisions more important than the

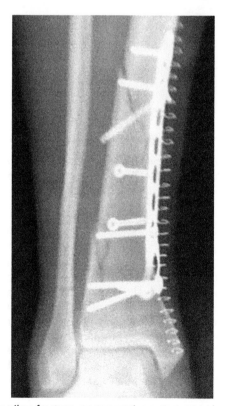

Fig. 13. Twisting injury pilon fracture, postoperative anteroposterior view.

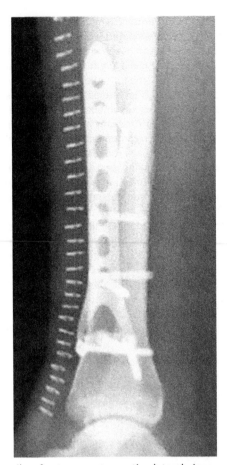

Fig. 14. Twisting injury pilon fracture, postoperative lateral view.

absolute distance between two incisions." Incisions should be kept small and should be straight to bone, to form full thickness flaps with limited periosteal stripping, to prevent devascularization of bone fragments (**Figs. 11–14**).[17]

External Fixation

In their randomized prospective study, Wyrsch and colleagues[35] compared the results of ORIF of both the tibia and fibula with the results of external fixation with or without limited internal fixation. These investigators concluded that, "external fixation is a satisfactory method of treatment for fractures of the tibial plafond and is associated with fewer complications than internal fixation." External fixation is most valuable as an adjunct treatment in severe pilon fractures with soft tissue compromise, because it limits the insult to the soft tissues, stabilizes the fracture to prevent further damage to the soft tissues, reestablishes limb length, and allows access for wound care.[5,26,29,77,92,93] The types of external fixators used include joint-spanning rigid, joint-spanning articulated, and nonjoint-spanning.[29,45,92,94–96] Marsh and colleagues[97] carried out a study comparing early motion and no motion using an articulated, joint-spanning fixator. Their results showed no significant difference in range of motion, Medical Outcomes Study 36-Item Short Form (SF-36) score, or ankle osteoarthritis scale. Another recent literature review comparing complication and union rates in joint-spanning and nonjoint-spanning external fixation in pilon fractures showed no significant difference in the rates of infection, nonunion, or time to union. However, the patients with joint-spanning external fixators did show a higher rate of malunion.[98]

Vidyadhara and Rao[60] proposed that Ilizarov external ring fixation "preserves endosteal and periosteal blood supply, helps capture the small metaphyseal and subchondral bony fragments, and also helps compression of fracture fragments using the olive wires" and that "It also allows correction of deformity during the process of fracture healing." These investigators also propose that the ring fixator can be used to achieve arthrodiastasis. Fortin[62] states that external fixation used alone "can result in less than anatomic reduction of the articular surface." Sanders and Stewart[16] propose and Thordarson[99] agrees that "It is our experience that the use of an external fixator as the sole treatment modality is associated with a high incidence of metaphyseal nonunion, or varus collapse resulting in tibial malunion." Pugh and colleagues[100] undertook a retrospective study of union rates after ORIF, joint-spanning external fixation, and hybrid external fixation performed within 6 days of injury. They found no significant difference in minor or major complication rates, but the rate of malunion was significantly lower in the ORIF group. However, Anglen[42] found that hybrid external fixation showed a significantly higher rate of nonunion and complications, and worse outcomes, than did ORIF, with no difference in the articular reduction. Fractures that are amenable to external fixation alone include those fractures with large articular fragments, open fractures with extensive soft tissue damage and metaphyseal comminution.[62] Because of the lack of rigid internal fixation, these fractures take longer to consolidate, and the patient may need to remain in the fixator, either weight bearing or nonweight bearing, for up to 4 months or more.[85,88]

Preferred Method

To date, the most effective treatment of complex pilon fractures, with the lowest risk of postoperative complications, is a staged approach involving early open reduction of the fibular fracture (if present) with application of an external fixator for temporary reduction and stabilization of the tibial fracture, followed by delayed, definitive, limited ORIF of the tibial fractures.

Nast-Kolb and colleagues[101] compared tibial plating with limited ORIF in pilon fractures and found that delayed union was twice as likely with tibial plating, and had a 2.5 times greater incidence of severe posttraumatic arthrosis. In 1993, Tornetta and colleagues[8] proposed a solution to these poor results: limited internal and hybrid external fixation. The results of this combination approach were anatomic reduction of the fractures and early functional results comparable with ORIF, without the soft tissue-related complications.

In 1956, Gay[2,3,5,7,9,37,66,77,102] were the first to recognize that stabilization of the fibula lead to alignment and reduction of the tibial articular surface, and fixation of the fibula is now the classic first step in treatment of pilon fractures. Tile[7] put it succinctly in 1987, "failure to reconstruct the fibula at all is a major error in judgment and may jeopardize the tibial reconstruction, as the tendency of the ankle to drift into valgus will be difficult to overcome."

The first step in surgical planning is evaluation of radiographs and CT scans in preparation of a surgical template. Incision planning before the initial fibular ORIF and external fixator placement is crucial. If the fracture is open, the traumatic wounds should be incorporated into the surgical incisions, if possible, especially if subsequent flap coverage is planned.[103] The fibular ORIF should be approached through a posterolateral incision, with care taken to avoid the peroneal nerve, so that there is a sufficient skin bridge left for the proposed tibial incision. Placement of a fibular plate can lead to prominent hardware and complaints from the patient.[104] The senior author (DMM) recommends consideration of fibular rod placement, such as the Acumed (Hillsboro, OR, USA) fibular intramedullary rod, in amenable fracture patterns, because this limits soft tissue disruption to small stab incisions at the distal lateral malleolus and for percutaneous screw placement. If tibial incisions or wounds are present, the lateral, fibular incision may be packed open to allow closure of the more crucial tibial incisions/wounds. External fixators should be placed so that the pins or wires do not interfere with the eventual incisions. The fixator itself can be used intraoperatively to aid in fracture reduction (**Figs. 15–20**).[103]

Analyzing the type of injury force involved in the fracture at hand helps to plan incision location and subsequent hardware placement. Valgus injury forces cause a comminuted, compression fracture of the fibula with a corresponding valgus fracture pattern in the tibia. These fractures are best served with lateral plating to withstand the valgus forces.[18] An anterolateral or Bohler incision can be used to access both the fibular fracture and the distal tibia, providing excellent exposure to the articular surface, the lateral column of the tibia, and the syndesmosis, as well as sufficient soft tissue coverage of any hardware.[105] Care must be taken to avoid the superficial peroneal nerve and the anterior perforating peroneal artery.[41]

Varus injury forces cause simple tension fractures of the fibula. The tibia is also in a varus alignment, and medially placed plates resist any further varus deformation.[18] The anteromedial approach to the distal tibia is common and provides good exposure to the central and medial articular surface and the medial column of the tibia, but less than optimal exposure of the lateral plafond or syndesmosis. This lack of access to the syndesmosis is most notable when the lateral tibial plafond (Chaput tubercle area) is

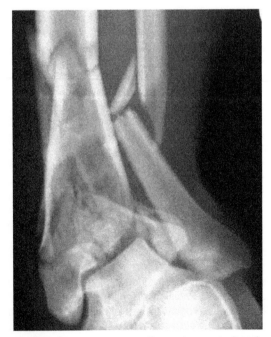

Fig. 15. High-energy pilon fracture, preoperative anteroposterior view. Patient jumped from a second- story window.

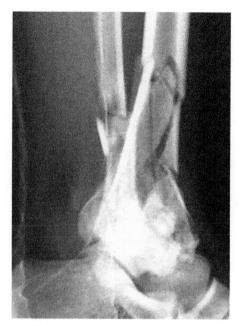

Fig. 16. High-energy pilon fracture, preoperative lateral view. Note the significant metaphyseal and articular comminution.

disconnected from the fibula, thus making reduction of the anterolateral fracture fragment by ligamentotaxis impossible. Patients also commonly complain of prominent, uncomfortable anteromedial hardware.[41]

In the more complex, significantly impacted plafond fractures, the articular surface may have little bony connection to the remaining tibial shaft, because of impaction of

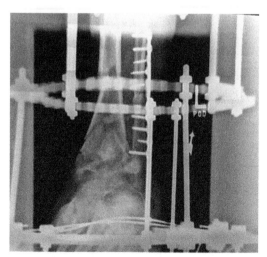

Fig. 17. High-energy pilon fracture, postoperative anteroposterior view. Preliminary external fixation and ORIF of fibula.

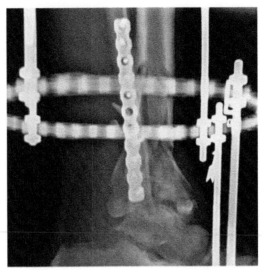

Fig. 18. High-energy pilon fracture, postoperative lateral view. Preliminary external fixation and ORIF of fibula.

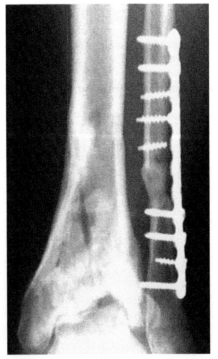

Fig. 19. Postoperative anteroposterior view of previous external fixation and fibular ORIF. Patient was incarcerated and lost to follow-up; therefore, staged reconstruction of articular surface and metaphyseal grafting never performed.

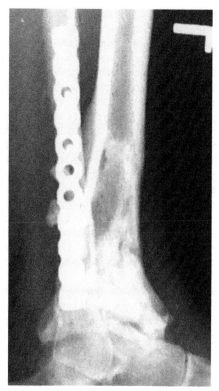

Fig. 20. Postoperative lateral view of previous external fixation and fibular ORIF. Patient was incarcerated and lost to follow-up; therefore, staged reconstruction of articular surface and metaphyseal grafting never performed.

the metaphyseal bone, so bone graft is required.[18] These fractures may require a straight anterior incisional approach, which may be used later for arthrodesis or total ankle replacement, if the articular surface is so severely comminuted as to be irreparable.[16,62]

Femino and colleagues[41] at the University of Iowa recommend an immediate repair of some pilon fractures with a single-incision lateral approach, at the posterolateral aspect of the fibula, which preserves the delicate soft tissue envelope at the anterior aspect of the ankle, the anterior tibial arterial blood supply, and protects the superficial peroneal nerve. Bhattacharyya and colleagues[106] also described a posterolateral approach and recommended limiting this approach to fractures with primarily posterior involvement, and in cases in which an anterior approach is precluded. This approach differs from the single lateral approach described by Grose and colleagues,[107] which lies along the anterior border of the fibula, offering poor visualization of the medial tibial plafond.

TECHNIQUE

As mentioned earlier, the senior author (DMM) advocates a staged procedure involving: (1) immediate irrigation and debridement of open wounds using standard open fracture protocol, (2) ORIF of the fibula through a posterolateral approach, or preferably fibular intramedullary rodding where applicable, through a stab incision, (3) application of external fixation to help reestablish length, rotation, and axial alignment and reduce tibial fracture fragments via ligamentotaxis, (4) delayed limited ORIF of articular surface and tibial shaft fractures through MIPO/miniopen technique, using incisions appropriate for injury force and fracture location, and (5) extended nonweight bearing with early range of motion, if possible.

Anatomic reduction of the fibular fracture with satisfactory recreation of fibular length, rotation, and angulation is crucial in setting the stage for future tibial fracture reduction. One author (DMM) recommends the Acumed fibular intramedullary rod for stabilization of the fibular component in pilon fractures, because it involves minimal soft tissue disruption and adequate restoration of length. More complicated fibular fractures can be approached by MIPO and bridging plate techniques discussed in the article on ankle fracture by Denise M. Mandi elsewhere in this issue.

Placement of the external fixator must allow for later incision placement for tibial fixation.[62] Many investigators recommend CT evaluation only after preliminary reduction and stabilization by external fixator.[23,24,62,65] It is not uncommon for the external fixator to remain in place for 3 to 4 weeks, depending on the status of the soft tissues, before the next step is attempted.[62]

Once the soft tissues have sufficiently recovered from the initial trauma of the injury, edema has reduced, open wounds have been managed, and, some investigators argue, fracture blisters have resolved (Mandracchia and colleagues[10] and other investigators have operated through both intradermal and subdermal fracture blisters with no ill effects), the next stage in treatment can begin, namely, reduction of the tibial plafond articular surface. MIPO and minimally invasive percutaneous plate osteosynthesis use small incisions to restore mechanical axes, decrease iatrogenic tissue injury, and preserve fracture hematoma.[108] Borrelli and colleagues[109] performed a cadaver study of the blood supply of the distal tibia and found that percutaneous plating led to substantially less injury to the extraosseous blood supply. Incisions placed either

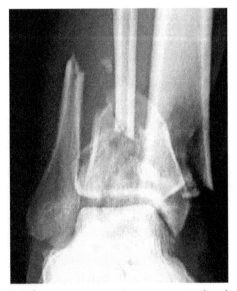

Fig. 21. High-energy pilon fracture, preoperative anteroposterior view.

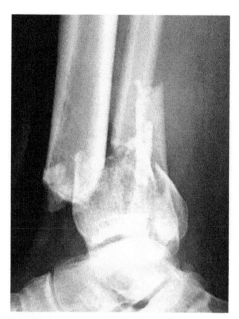

Fig. 22. High-energy pilon fracture, preoperative lateral view.

anterolaterally or anteromedially should be kept only large enough to allow access to the tibial plafond and larger tibial shaft fragments. In some cases, reestablishing the structure of the proximal tibial shaft aids in the reduction of the distal fractures.[10] Every attempt should be made to leave periosteal attachments intact, to preserve blood

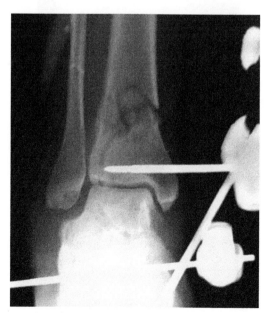

Fig. 23. High-energy pilon fracture, anteroposterior view, after preliminary external fixation.

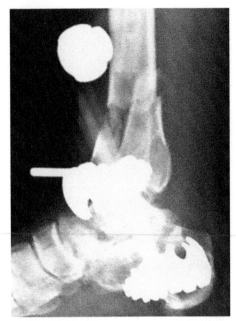

Fig. 24. High-energy pilon fracture, lateral view, after preliminary external fixation.

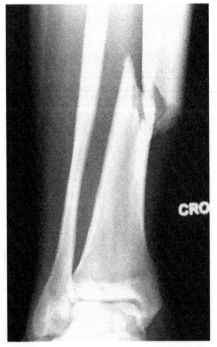

Fig. 25. Preoperative anteroposterior view of twisting pilon fracture, intra-articular extension difficult to see on this view.

supply and ligamentotaxis potential.[62] If the AITFL is still intact, then the anterolateral Chaput fragment acts as a reference point in the reduction of the plafond fracture.[62]

The articular surface fracture should be reduced from posterior to anterior and from lateral to medial, so that the deeper recesses of the joint are not obscured by premature fixation of the more superficial fragments. The anterior fracture fragments can be retracted aside, as in opening a book, to allow visualization of and access to the more posterior fracture fragments.[16,62] Typically, the medial malleolar fracture fragment is the last piece of the puzzle to be reduced, and it remains retracted for most of the operation.[16] Distraction across the joint at this point, by external fixator or other method, facilitates visualization of the joint surface.[62] The senior author (DMM) attempts to reduce the articular surface fragments and fixate them under compression using provisional K-wires followed by isolated lag screws and cut and buried K-wires as needed. We do not favor absorbable fixation because of the propensity for cystic formation surrounding these absorbable pins, which could be catastrophic near a joint surface. Some of these K-wires are inserted percutaneously, if adequate exposure is not available through the limited incision. All that is needed is a single plafond fragment in its original anatomic position (often the Volkmann or Chaput fragment) to act as the anchor to which all other fragments are attached. Larger articular fragments are separately lagged to the main anchor fragment, and smaller fragments are held in place by

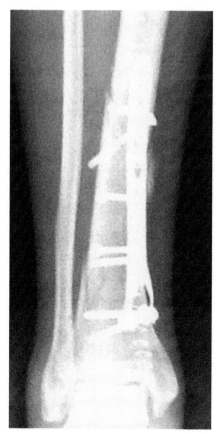

Fig. 26. Postoperative lateral view of same pilon fracture.

compression from surrounding fragments or K-wire (either temporary or buried).[16,110] Sommer and Ruedi[17] recommend that "All articular fragments are lined up one after the other using the talus as a mold to restore anatomic congruence." If there is a central articular defect or nonviable fragments (which must be removed), a lag screw can span the defect, maintaining the articular dimensions. The defect can then be grafted along with any metaphyseal defects.[17,111] Fortin[62] reminds us that "Articular malunion is the result of inadequate reduction and is very difficult to manage."

Once all viable articular fracture fragments have been reduced and fixated, this stable articular block or joint block is then connected to the proximal tibial shaft via screws (in pilon fractures without significant comminution) or by low profile plating. These plates should be used with minimal dissection and placed supraperiosteally via tunneling through the soft tissues and making small incisions to allow the plates to be pulled through the tunnel into place. The plate is then secured to the bone with percutaneous screws, to minimize soft tissue disruption. Alternatively, incisions for plate placement can be made overlying the fracture plane to minimize soft tissue stripping.[99] Some investigators recommend external fixation usage to avoid placement of large plates up the diaphysis on pilon fractures with significant proximal extension,[99] but we have found that placing a long plate, supraperiosteally, under nontraumatized soft tissue does not cause any significant compromise to the soft tissue.

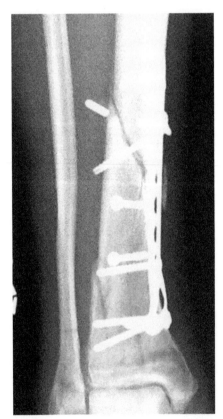

Fig. 27. First evidence of trouble: broken hardware caused by weight bearing against medical advice.

Recommended indications for locking plates in pilon fractures are small fracture fragments, comminution and osteoporosis, but minimal data exist supporting better outcomes with use of locking plates.[18,23] Yenna and colleagues[112] investigated anterolateral and medial locking plates in distal tibial fractures and found that "Distal tibial extra-articular fractures stabilized with anterolateral or medial locking plate constructs demonstrated no statistically significant difference in biomechanical stiffness in compression and torsion testing."

Once the plate is placed to stabilize the articular block to the shaft, any subchondral and metaphyseal defects should be bone grafted with either autogenous bone graft or bone substitute, taking care to avoid what is known as a dead bone sandwich.[17,110] If there is any concern about infection, or if bone graft is not available, any defect can be filled temporarily with antibiotic impregnated bone cement (as a block or beads).[110] Some investigators recommend arthroscopy to evaluate the condition of the articular surface or to aid in reduction of the articular fracture fragments. Although it may be helpful in reducing the plafond fracture, and is minimally invasive to the vulnerable soft tissues, it has not been proved to improve outcomes.[23]

When possible, closure of all incisions should be performed at the time of definitive ORIF. If significant soft tissue compromise (degloving, devascularization, crush) is present, or closure over implants/exposed bone is not possible, then muscle flaps or free flaps must be considered, better earlier than later.[110]

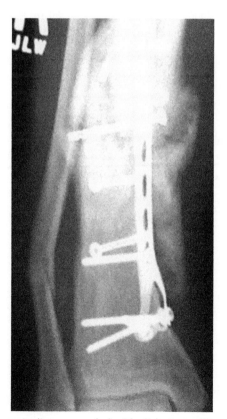

Fig. 28. Continuing noncompliance, coupled with diabetes mellitus, alcohol and nicotine abuse, cause continuing deformation and failure. Note patient-induced fibular fracture.

Perhaps the best advice concerning the management of pilon fractures comes from Sommer and Ruedi[17]: "Complex pilon fractures should therefore be treated by the most experienced surgeons and are not the domain of the junior staff" (**Figs. 21–24**).

POSTOPERATIVE CONSIDERATIONS AND COMPLICATIONS

The most common complications after pilon fracture are related to soft tissue. The high-energy nature of these fractures, coupled with the significant trauma to the soft tissue envelope, sets the stage for dehiscence, skin necrosis, and superficial infection in from 8% to 35% of patients. Deep infections are seen in 0% to 55% of cases. Delayed or nonunions are found in 0% to 22% and posttraumatic arthritis in 13% to 54% of pilon fractures. The literature reports that "There is almost a 100% correlation between deep infection and the subsequent need for ankle arthrodesis."[3,10,13,17,25,32,37,48,57,78,88,113]

Because soft tissue dictates the timing and type of surgical intervention, and most complications stem from the soft tissue, it makes sense to stack the deck in your favor regarding preservation of the soft tissue envelope during the postoperative period. Negative pressure wound therapy (NPWT) or wound vacs are commonly used in open wounds to remove drainage and stimulate granulation, and are certainly appropriate in treatment of open pilon fractures. Some advocate NPWT over surgical incisions, but this has not shown any significant benefit.[23] Atraumatic technique with careful tissue handling during surgery and good, basic wound care postoperatively,

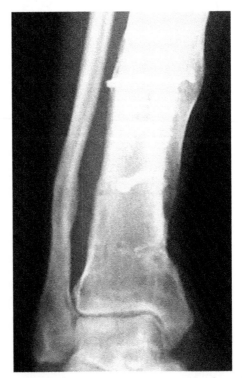

Fig. 29. After prolonged immobilization, and some cooperation from the patient, hardware was prominent, and eventually removed.

coupled with leaving sutures or staples in place for 3 to 4 weeks, until tissue healing is assured, helps to prevent some wound dehiscence.

Crist and colleagues[23] caution that "In general, it is easier to manage complications related to closed management (eg, malunion, arthrosis) than those related to ill-advised ORIF (eg, infection, wound breakdown)." If deep infection develops, it must be treated quickly and aggressively by debridement and appropriate intravenous antibiotics. Do not be too quick to remove hardware, even in the face of deep infection, until the fracture has healed or can be definitively stabilized by an external fixator.[16] The senior author (DMM) has found through bitter experience that it is easier to treat an infection in a healed fracture than it is to treat an infection and a displaced fracture. All necrotic fragments must be removed and antibiotic cement inserted in their place (**Figs. 25–29**).[16]

If there is anything that we have learned in the treatment of pilon fractures, it is "Never trust a tibia." The senior author (DMM) has seen pilon fractures that appeared consolidated across the fracture lines, as long as 8 months postoperatively, crumble and buckle with weight bearing. Megas and colleagues[114] reported that the nonunion rate in distal tibial fractures is the highest of all long bone fractures. Nonunions usually occur at the metaphyseal-diaphyseal junction because of traumatic devascularization, soft tissue stripping, and inadequate stabilization of the fracture fragments.[62] These nonunions often occur medially, causing varus malalignment.[62] Because of the tenuous blood supply in the diaphysis of the tibia, the traumatic damage to the surrounding support structures, and the comminution commonly seen in pilon

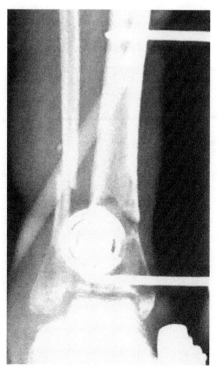

Fig. 30. Preliminary external fixation of pilon fracture, anteroposterior view. Patient remained nonweight bearing for 6 months, using external bone stimulator.

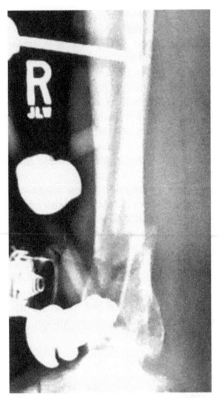

Fig. 31. Preliminary external fixation of pilon fracture, lateral view.

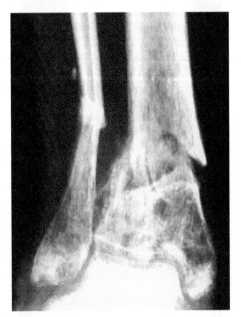

Fig. 32. After removal of external fixator, anteroposterior view. Patient walked on the leg, against medical advice, 7 months after injury.

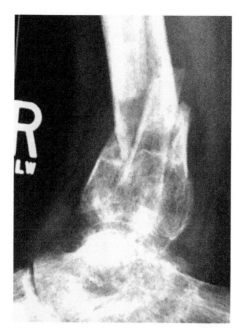

Fig. 33. After removal of external fixator, lateral view. Note significant sagittal plane deformity secondary to patient's weight bearing against medical advice.

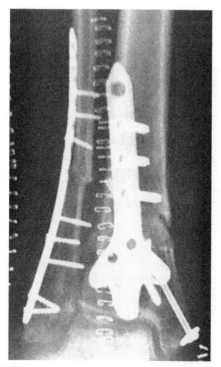

Fig. 34. Pilon fracture failure, anteroposterior view, status post osteotomy, bone grafting, and ORIF.

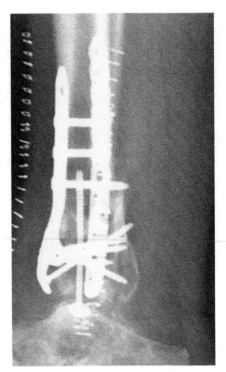

Fig. 35. Pilon fracture failure, lateral view, status post osteotomy, bone grafting, and ORIF.

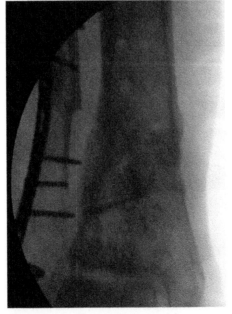

Fig. 36. Prominent hardware eventually required removal.

fractures, it is prudent to delay weight bearing until bony union is certain: various investigators recommend from 3 to 8 months nonweight bearing or partial weight bearing (**Figs. 30–36**).[10,18,111]

SUMMARY

The nature of the pilon fracture has caused evolution of our treatment methods and its historically high rate of complication and poor outcome continue to direct our choice of treatment.[23] Results after pilon fracture are tied to the initial injury, its severity, mechanism, displacement, and force. Although anatomic reduction and stable fixation allow early motion after pilon fracture, stiffness is still a common result. Anatomic reduction does not guarantee a good result.[99] Thus, pilon fractures are not only challenging for the surgeon, but can be frustrating as well. Long-term follow-up of patients surgically treated for pilon fractures shows that degenerative joint disease occurs in most patients, even after anatomic reduction of the joint surface, most likely because of the severe initial damage to the cartilaginous surfaces at the time of injury.[62,111] Patient satisfaction and functional outcome do not always reflect what is seen on the radiograph.[62] Pilon fracture outcomes are dependent on so many factors, they can be difficult to predict.[23] Preparing the patient mentally is nearly as important as preparing them physically, so that their expectations for function after the injury are realistic.

REFERENCES

1. Destot E. Traumatismes du pied et rayons X malleoles: astragale, calcanetun, avantipied. Paris: Masson; 1911.
2. Bone LB. Fractures of the tibial plafond: the pilon fracture. Orthop Clin North Am 1987;18:95–104.
3. Kellam JF, Waddell JP. Fractures of the distal tibial metaphysis with intra-articular extension: the distal explosion fracture. J Trauma 1979;19:593–601.
4. Ovadia DN, Beals RK. Fractures of the tibial plafond. J Bone Joint Surg Am 1986;68:543–51.
5. Ruedi TP. Fractures of the lower end of the tibia into the ankle joint: results 9 years after open reduction and internal fixation. Injury 1973;5:130–4.
6. Ruedi TP, Allgower M. Fractures of the lower end of the tibia into the ankle joint. Injury 1969;1(2):92–9.
7. Tile M. Fractures of the distal tibial metaphysis involving the ankle joint: the pilon fracture. In: Schatzker J, Tile M, editors. The rationale of operative fracture care. Berlin: Springer-Verlag; 1987. p. 343–69.
8. Tornetta P, Weiner LS, Bergman M, et al. Pilon fractures: treatment with combined internal and external fixation. J Orthop Trauma 1993;7:489–96.
9. Trafton PG, Bray TJ, Simpson LA. Fractures and soft-tissue injuries of the ankle. In: Browner BD, Jupiter JB, Levine AM, et al, editors. Skeletal Trauma, vol. 2. Philadelphia: WB Saunders; 1992. p. 1931–41.
10. Mandracchia VJ, Evans RD, Nelson SC, et al. Pilon fractures of the distal tibia. Clin Podiatr Med Surg 1999;16:743–67.
11. Bonin JG. Injuries to the ankle. London: William Heinemann; 1950. 248–60.
12. Kelikian H, Kelikian A. Pilon fractures. In: Kelikian H, Kelikian A, editors. Disorders of the ankle. Philadelphia: WB Saunders; 1985. p. 569–607.
13. Teeny SM, Wiss DA. Open reduction and internal fixation of tibial plafond fractures: variables contribution to poor results and complications. Clin Orthop 1993;292:108–17.

14. Bartlett CS, D'Amato MJ, Weiner LS. Fractures of the tibial pilon in skeletal trauma: fractures, dislocations, and ligamentous injuries. In: Browner BD, Jupiter JB, Levine AM, et al, editors. Skeletal trauma, vol. 2. Philadelphia: WB Saunders; 1998. p. 2295–325.

15. Pollack AN, McMarthy ML, Bess RS, et al. Outcomes after treatment of high-energy tibial plafond fractures. J Bone Joint Surg 2003;85(10):1893–900.

16. Sanders R, Stewart JD. Tibial periarticular fractures reduction and fixation. In: Kitaoka HB, editor. Master techniques in orthopaedic surgery: the foot and ankle. 2nd edition. Philadelphia: Lippincott Williams & Wilkins; 2002. p. 631–42.

17. Sommer C, Ruedi TP. Tibia: distal (pilon). In: Ruedi TP, Murphy WM, Colton CL, et al, editors. AO principles of fracture management. Stuttgart (Germany), NY: Thieme; 2000. p. 543–60.

18. Sirkin MS. Plating of tibial pilon fractures. Am J Orthop 2007;36(Suppl 12):13–7.

19. Muller ME, Allgower M, Schneider R, et al. Manual of internal fixation: techniques recommended by the AO Group. 2nd editon. New York: Springer-Verlag; 1979. p. 146–7, 208–10, 214–5, 586–612.

20. Muller ME, Nazarian S, Koch P, et al. Comprehensive classification of fractures of long bones. New York: Springer-Verlag; 1987. p. 170–9.

21. Craig S, Bartlett C, Lon S, et al. Fracture of the tibial pilon. In: Browner B, Jupiter J, Levine A, et al, editors. Skeletal trauma. 3rd edition. Singapore: Elsevier; 2003. p. 2257.

22. McMillen RL, Gruen GS. Advancements in percutaneous fixation for foot and ankle trauma. Clin Podiatr Med Surg 2011;28:711–26.

23. Crist BD, Khazzam M, Murtha YM, et al. Pilon fractures: advances in surgical management. J Am Acad Orthop Surg 2011;19:612–22.

24. Topliss CJ, Jackson M, Atkins RM. Anatomy of pilon fractures of the distal tibia. J Bone Joint Surg Br 2005;87:692–7.

25. Heim U. The pilon tibial fracture: classification, surgical techniques, results. Philadelphia: WB Saunders; 1995.

26. Mast JW, Spiegal PG, Pappas JN. Fractures of tibial pilon. Clin Orthop 1988; 230:68–82.

27. Waddell JP. Tibial plafond fractures. In: Tscherne H, Schatzker J, editors. Major fractures of the pilon, the talus, and the calcaneus. Heidelberg (Germany): Springer-Verlag; 1993. p. 43–8.

28. Yablon IG, Segal D, Leach RE. Ankle injuries. New York: Churchill Livingstone; 1983.

29. Bone L, Stegemann P, McNamara K, et al. External fixation of severely comminuted and open tibial pilon fractures. Clin Orthop Relat Res 1993;292: 101–7.

30. Saleh M, Shanahan MD, Fern ED. Intra-articular fractures of the distal tibia: surgical management by limited internal fixation and articulated distraction. Injury 1993;24:37–40.

31. Sirkin M, Sanders R, DiPasquale T, et al. A staged protocol for soft tissue management in the treatment of complex pilon fractures. J Orthop Trauma 1999;13:78–84.

32. McFerran MA, Smith SW, Boulas HJ, et al. Complications encountered in the treatment of pilon fractures. J Orthop Trauma 1992;6:195–200.

33. Pierce RO Jr, Heinrich JH. Comminuted intra-articular fractures of the distal tibia. J Trauma 1979;19:828–32.

34. Sands A, Grujic L, Byck DC, et al. Clinical and functional outcomes of internal fixation of displaced pilon fractures. Clin Orthop Relat Res 1998;347:131–7.

35. Wyrsch B, McFerran MA, McAndrew M, et al. Operative treatment of fractures of the tibial plafond. A randomized, prospective study. J Bone Joint Surg Am 1996; 78:1646–57.

36. Sanders R, Pappas J, Mast J, et al. The salvage of open grade IIIB ankle and talus fractures. J Orthop Trauma 1992;6:201–8.

37. Bourne RB. Pylon fractures of the distal tibia. Clin Orthop Relat Res 1989;240: 42–6.

38. Patterson MJ, Cole JD. Two-staged delayed open reduction and internal fixation of severe pilon fractures. J Orthop Trauma 1999;13(2):85–91.

39. Blauth M, Bastian L, Krettek C, et al. Surgical options for the treatment of severe tibial pilon fractures: a study of three techniques. J Orthop Trauma 2001;15(3): 153–60.

40. Borrelli J Jr, Catalano L. Open reduction and internal fixation of pilon fractures. J Orthop Trauma 1999;13(8):573–82.

41. Femino JE, Vaseenon T. The direct lateral approach to the distal tibia and fibula: a single incision technique for distal tibial and pilon fractures. Iowa Orthop J 2010;29:143–8.

42. Anglen JO. Early outcome of hybrid external fixation for fracture of the distal tibia. J Orthop Trauma 1999;13(2):92–7.

43. Beck E. Results of operative treatment of pilon fractures. In: Tscherne H, Schatzker J, editors. Major fractures of the pilon, the talus, and calcaneus. Heidelberg (Germany): Springer-Verlag; 1993. p. 49–51.

44. Helfet DL, Koval K, Pappas J, et al. Intra-articular pilon fractures of the tibia. Clin Orthop 1994;298:221–8.

45. Karas E, Weiner L. Displaced pilon fractures: an update. Orthop Clin North Am 1994;25:651–63.

46. Ruwe PA, Randall RL, Baumgaertner MR. Pilon fractures of the distal tibia. Orthop Rev 1993;22:987–96.

47. Metcalfe BP. Pilon fractures of the tibia. Curr Orthop 2003;17(3):190–9.

48. Dillin L, Slabaugh P. Delayed wound healing, infection, and nonunion following open reduction and internal fixation of tibial plafond fractures. J Trauma 1986; 26(12):1116–9.

49. Watson JT, Moed BR, Karges DE, et al. Pilon fractures: treatment protocol based on severity of soft tissue injury. Clin Orthop Relat Res 2000;(375):78–90.

50. Conroy J, Agarwal M, Giannoudis PV, et al. Early internal fixation and soft tissue cover of severe open tibial pilon fractures. Int Orthop 2003;27(6):343–7.

51. Trentz O, Friedl HP. Critical soft-tissue conditions in pilon fractures. In: Tscherne H, Schatzker J, editors. Major fractures of the pilon, the talus, and the calcaneus. Berlin, Heidelberg, New York: Springer-Verlag; 1993. p. 59–64.

52. Rommens PM, Claes P, DeBoodt P, et al. Therapeutic procedure and long-term results in tibial pilon fracture in relation to primary soft-tissue damage. Unfallchirurg 1994;97(1):39–46.

53. Crutchfield EH, Seligson D, Henry SL, et al. Tibial pilon fractures: a comparative clinical study of management techniques and results. Orthopedics 1995;18(7): 613–7.

54. McDonald MG, Burgess RC, Bolano LE, et al. Ilizarov treatment of pilon fractures. Clin Orthop 1996;(325):232–8.

55. Leonard M, Magill P, Khayyat G. Minimally-invasive treatment of high velocity intra-articular fractures of the distal tibia. Int Orthop 2009;33(4):1149–53.

56. Borrelli J Jr, Ellis E. Pilon fractures: assessment and treatment. Orthop Clin North Am 2002;33:231–45.

57. Bourne RB, Horabeck CH, MacNab BA. Intra-articular fractures of the distal tibia: the pilon fracture. J Trauma 1983;23:591–6.
58. Etter C, Ganz R. Long-term results of tibial plafond fractures treated with open reduction and internal fixation. Arch Orthop Trauma Surg 1991;110:277–83.
59. Helfet DL, Shonnard PY, Levine D, et al. Minimally invasive plate osteosynthesis of distal fractures of the tibia. Injury 1997;28(Suppl):SA42–8.
60. Vidyadhara S, Rao SK. Ilizarov treatment of complex tibial pilon fractures. Int Orthop 2006;30(2):113–7.
61. White TO, Guy P, Cooke CJ, et al. The results of early primary open reduction and internal fixation for treatment of OTA 43.C-type tibial pilon fractures: a cohort study. J Orthop Trauma 2010;24(12):757–63.
62. Fortin PT. Pilon fractures in advanced reconstruction–foot and ankle. In: Nunley JA, Pfeffer GB, Sanders RW, et al, editors. Advanced reconstruction foot & ankle. Rosemont (IL): American Academy of Orthopaedic Surgeons; 2004. p. 363–8.
63. Wagner HE, Jakob RP. Plate osteosynthesis in bicondylar fractures of the tibial head. Unfallchirurg 1986;89(7):304–11.
64. Webb LX, Birkedal J, Nierengarten MB. Open tibial pilon fractures: complications and issues of limb salvage. Medscape Orthop 2001;5(3) [online].
65. Tornetta P III, Gorup J. Axial computed tomography of pilon fractures. Clin Orthop 1996;(323):273–6.
66. Gay R, Evrard J. Les fractures recentes du pilon tibial chez l'adulte. Rev Chir Orthop 1963;49:397–512.
67. Ayeni JP. Pilon fractures of the tibia: a study based on 19 cases. Injury 1988;19: 109–14.
68. Braustein PW, Wade PA. Treatment of unstable fractures of the ankle. Ann Surg 1959;149:217–26.
69. Burwell HN, Charnley AD. The treatment of displaced fractures of the ankle by rigid internal fixation and early joint movement. J Bone Joint Surg Br 1965;47: 634–60.
70. Coonrad RW. Fracture-dislocations of the ankle joint with impaction injury to the lateral weight bearing surface of the tibia. J Bone Joint Surg Am 1970;52: 1337–43.
71. Jergesen F. Open reduction of fractures and dislocations of the ankle. Am J Surg 1959;98:136.
72. Klossner O. Late results of operative and nonoperative treatment of severe ankle fractures. Acta Chir Scand Suppl 1962;293:1–93.
73. Lauge-Hansen N. Fractures of the ankle: pronation-dorsiflexion fractures. Arch Surg 1953;67(pt 5):813–20.
74. Leach RE. A means of stabilizing comminuted distal tibial fractures. J Trauma 1964;4:722–5.
75. MacKinnon AP. Fracture of the lower articular surface of the tibia in fracture dislocation of the ankle. J Bone Joint Surg Am 1928;10:352.
76. Marsh JL, Bonar S, Nepola JV, et al. Use of an articulated external fixator for fractures of the tibial plafond. J Bone Joint Surg 1995;774:1498–509.
77. Mast JW, Jacobs R, Ganz R. Planning and reduction techniques in fracture surgery. Berlin: Springer-Verlag; 1989. p. 182–4.
78. Moller BN, Krebs B. Intra-articular fractures of the distal tibia. Acta Orthop Scand 1982;53:991–6.
79. Picanza J. Poor results mark ORIF of tibial plafond fractures. Orthop Today 1990;10:1.

80. Treadwell JR, Fallat LM. Dynamic unilateral distraction fixation: surgical management of tibial pilon fractures. J Foot Ankle Surg 1994;33:438–42.
81. Varela CD, Vaughan TK, Carr JB, et al. Fracture blisters: clinical and pathological aspects. J Orthop Trauma 1993;7:417–27.
82. Maale G, Seligson D. Fractures through the distal weight-bearing surface of the tibia. Orthopedics 1980;3:507–12.
83. VanderGriend R, Michelson JD, Bone LB. Fractures of the ankle and distal part of the tibia. J Bone Joint Surg Am 1993;78:1772–83.
84. Cox FJ. Fractures of the ankle involving the lower articular surface of the tibia. Clin Orthop 1965;42:51–5.
85. Murphy CP, D'Ambrosia R, Dabezies EJ. The small pin circular fixator for distal tibial pilon fractures with soft-tissue compromise. Orthopedics 1991;14: 283–90.
86. Franklin JL, Johnson KD, Hansen ST. Immediate internal fixation of open ankle fractures: report of 38 cases treated with a standard protocol. J Bone Joint Surg Am 1984;66:1349–56.
87. Gustilo RB, Anderson JT. Prevention of infection in the treatment of 1025 open fractures of the long bones: retrospective and prospective analysis. J Bone Joint Surg Am 1976;58:453–8.
88. Leone VJ, Ruland R, Meinhard B. The management of soft tissue in pilon fractures. Clin Orthop 1993;292:315–20.
89. Fogel GR, Morrey BF. Delayed open reduction and fixation of ankle fractures. Clin Orthop 1987;215:187.
90. Muller KH, Presscher W. Post-traumatische Osteomyelitis nach distalen intra-articularen Unterschenkelfrakturen. Hefte Unfallheilkd 1978;131:163–83.
91. Muller ME. Les fractures du pilon tibial. Rev Chir Orthop 1964;50:557.
92. Ries MD, Meinhard BP. Medial external fixation with lateral plate internal fixation in metaphyseal tibia fractures: a report of eight cases with severe soft-tissue injury. Clin Orthop 1990;256:215–24.
93. Ruedi T, Allgower M. The operative treatment of intra-articular fractures of the lower end of the tibia. Clin Orthop 1979;138:105–10.
94. Barbieri R, Schenk RS, Aurori KC, et al. Hybrid external fixation in the treatment of tibial pilon fractures. Presented at the 11th Annual Meeting of the Orthopaedic Trauma Association. Tampa (FL), September, 1995.
95. Collins DN, Temple SD. Open joint injuries. Clin Orthop 1989;243:48–56.
96. DiChristina D, Riemer B, Butterfield S, et al. Pilon fractures treated with an articulated external fixator: a preliminary report of significant complications. Presented at the 9th Annual Meeting of the Orthopaedic Trauma Association. New Orleans (LA), September, 1993.
97. Marsh JL, Muehling V, Dirschl D, et al. Tibial plafond fractures treated by articulated external fixation: a randomized trial of postoperative motion versus non-motion. J Orthop Trauma 2006;20(8):536–41.
98. Bacon S, Smith WR, Morgan SJ, et al. A retrospective analysis of comminuted intra-articular fractures of the tibial plafond: open reduction and internal fixation versus external Ilizarov fixation. Injury 2008;39(2):196–202.
99. Thordarson DB. Foot and ankle trauma. In: Thordarson DB, editor. Foot and ankle. Philadelphia: Lippincott Williams & Wilkins; 2004. p. 288–97.
100. Pugh KJ, Wolinshy PR, McAndrew MP, et al. Tibial pilon fractures: a comparison of treatment methods. J Trauma 1999;47(5):937–41.
101. Nast-Kolb D, Betz A, Rodel C, et al. Minimal osteosynthesis of the tibial pilon fracture. Unfallchirurg 1993;96:517–23.

102. Allgower M, Muller ME, Willenegger HT. Teknik der Operativen Frakturbehandlung. New York: Springer-Verlag; 1963.
103. Boraiah S, Kemp TJ, Erwteman A, et al. Outcome following open reduction and internal fixation of open pilon fractures. J Bone Joint Surg Am 2010;92:346–52.
104. Williams TM, Marsh JL, Nepola JV, et al. External fixation of tibial plafond fractures: is routine plating of the fibula necessary? J Orthop Trauma 1998;12(1): 16–20.
105. Herscovici D Jr, Sanders RW, Infante A, et al. Bohler incision: an extensile anterolateral approach to the foot and ankle. J Orthop Trauma 2000;14(6):429–32.
106. Bhattacharyya T, Crichlow R, Gobezie R, et al. Complications associated with the posterolateral approach for pilon fractures. J Orthop Trauma 2006;20(2): 104–7.
107. Grose A, Gardner MJ, Hettrich C, et al. Open reduction and internal fixation of tibial pilon fractures using a lateral approach. J Orthop Trauma 2007;21(8): 530–7.
108. Krettek C, Schandelmaier P, Miclau T, et al. Minimally invasive percutaneous plate osteosynthesis (MIPPO) using the DCS in proximal and distal femoral fractures. Injury 1997;28(Suppl 1):A20–30.
109. Borrelli J Jr, Prickett W, Song E, et al. Extraosseous blood supply of the tibia and the effects of different plating techniques: a human cadaveric study. J Orthop Trauma 2002;16(10):691–5.
110. Hessman M, Nork S, Sommer C, et al. Fixation of complex pilon fracture through anteromedial approach. In: Trafton P, editor. AO surgery reference. Davos, Switzerland: AO Foundation; 2011. p. 1–13.
111. Geissler WB, Tsao AK, Hughes JL. Fractures of the ankle. In: Rockwood CA, Green DP, Bucholz RW, et al, editors. Fractures in adults. 4th edition. Philadelphia: Lippincott-Raven; 1996. p. 2202–66.
112. Yenna ZC, Bhadra AK, Ojike NI, et al. Anterolateral and medial locking plate stiffness in distal tibial fracture model. Foot Ankle Int 2011;6:630–6.
113. Cierny G, Byrd HS, Jones RE. Primary versus delayed soft-tissue coverage for severe open tibial fractures. Clin Orthop 1983;178:54–63.
114. Megas P, Zouboulis P, Papadopoulos AX. Distal tibial fractures and nonunions treated with shortened intramedullary nail. Int Orthop 2003;27:348–51.

Overview of Concepts and Treatments in Open Fractures

Nicole Jedlicka, DPM[a], N. Jake Summers, BS[b],
Mica M. Murdoch, DPM[c],*

KEYWORDS

• Open fracture • Treatment • Surgery • Emergency

Surgical emergencies related to the lower extremities are typically related to incidence of compartment syndrome, gas gangrene, septic joints, and open fractures. An open fracture is when osseous injuries disrupt and penetrate the skin, resulting in exposure of the fracture to the open environment, usually accompanied by injuries of varying severity to the soft tissue.[1] It has been estimated that between 3.5 million and 6 million fractures occur every year in the United States, approximately 3% of which are classified as open fractures.[2–4] This article reviews the current concepts used to manage and treat open fractures of the lower extremity and reviews treatment recommendations currently available in the literature. Typical concepts include classification, initial treatment and evaluation, antibiotic use, debridement and irrigation, timing of surgical treatment and wound closure, and stabilization of the injury.

INITIAL EVALUATION AND TREATMENT GOALS

Initial evaluation of open fractures should include a complete trauma work-up with considerations for hemorrhage, shock, neurovascular compromise, and tetanus immunization/prophylaxis. Other initial steps might also include laboratory studies, radiographs, and computed tomography, magnetic resonance imaging, or ultrasound as deemed necessary by the emergency room and surgeon.[5] Zwipp[6] created a list of priorities when dealing with soft tissue trauma. These include immediate soft tissue release, urgent release of compartment syndrome, primary partial amputation, second-look and third-look procedures in the OR, early soft tissue repair, choosing optimal surgical procedures, minimizing surgeon-related trauma, minimizing hardware

[a] Covenant Medical Center, Waterloo, IA 50702, USA
[b] Collage of Podiatric Medicine and Surgery, Des Moines University, 3200 Grand Avenue, Des Moines, IA 50312, USA
[c] Broadlawns Medical Center, 1801 Hickman Road, Des Moines, IA 50314, USA
* Corresponding author.
E-mail address: mmurdoch@broadlawns.org

Clin Podiatr Med Surg 29 (2012) 279–290
doi:10.1016/j.cpm.2012.01.006
0891-8422/12/$ – see front matter © 2012 Published by Elsevier Inc.

in complex trauma, using gentle distraction for reduction, and facilitating wound care and temporary external fixation.[6,7]

Gustilo[8] developed the following 8 principles that he thought essential in the treatment of open fractures. (1) All open fractures should be treated as surgical emergencies. (2) The patient should be evaluated for other life-threatening injuries. Most open fractures occur with multiple or severe trauma and high-energy accidents like motor vehicle accidents. (3) Appropriate and adequate antibiotic therapy is begun. (4) Appropriate irrigation and debridement is performed. (5) The open fracture should be stabilized. (6) Wound healing should be considered. (7) Early cancellous bone grafting should be performed. (8) Rehabilitation should be begun as early in the recovery process as possible (**Box 1**).[8]

Prophylactic treatment with tetanus immunization therapy should be considered for every patient with an open fracture. Also, puncture wounds, crush injuries, burns, frostbite, or wounds possibly contaminated with feces, dirt, or saliva should be highly suspicious for the presence of *Clostridium tetani*.[9] The Center for Disease Control recommends immunization with tetanus toxoids in any patient with an open fracture, or who has not had the immunization or a booster within the last 5 years. It is recommended that this toxoid is combined with the human tetanus immune globulin for any wounds showing suspicion of colonization with *C tetani*, immunocompromised individuals, or in patients not having had a booster in the past 10 years.[9]

CLASSIFICATIONS

The National Research Council in 1964 classified 4 types of wounds based on the risk of infection: (1) clean, (2) clean-contaminated, (3) contaminated, and (4) dirty. Open fractures are in the contaminated or dirty categories.[10] Any traumatic wound that is less than 4 hours old is considered by the council to be contaminated. These wounds have an infection rate of 20%. Dirty wounds have devitalized tissues, foreign bodies, or are greater than 4 hours old. Infection rate is between 28% and 70%.[10]

The Gustilo and Anderson[11] Classification of Open Fractures is the most widely accepted method of classification, and contains subsequent modifications. In this system, open fractures are classified as 1 of 3 types relative to the mechanism of injury, soft tissue damage, level of contamination, and degree of skeletal involvement.[11–13]

- Type 1: open fractures characterized as those with a wound that is less than 1 cm in length, and clean. There is minimal soft tissue injury and no crushing-type injury. The fracture associated with these types of wounds is typically a simple fracture, inside to outside, with minimal or no comminution.

Box 1
Gustillo[8] principles of open fracture management

- All open fractures are surgical emergencies
- Evaluate patient for other life-threatening injuries
- Use appropriate and adequate antibiotic therapy
- Perform appropriate irrigation and debridement
- Stabilize fracture
- Consider wound healing
- Cancellous bone grafting should be performed early
- Rehabilitation should begin early

- Type 2: open fractures with a laceration that is more than 1 cm in length. There is moderate soft tissue compromise and contamination. The fracture associated with these types of wounds shows moderate comminution and can be either of simple transverse or short oblique configurations.
- Type 3: open fractures accompanied by extensive soft tissue damage to the muscle, skin, and neurovascular structures. There is severe soft tissue compromise associated with a crushing component or a high-velocity injury (ie, gunshot wounds, farm injuries, amputations, car accidents, open fractures more than 8 hours old). The fractures associated with these types of wounds usually show severe comminution and displacement (**Fig. 1**).[11]
  - Type 3A: shows extensive laceration but adequate soft tissue coverage and severe comminution.
  - Type 3B: shows extensive soft tissue loss, periosteal stripping and bone exposure with large amounts of contamination and comminution.
  - Type 3C: shows an open fracture with arterial injury with the highest potential for infection and complication.[12]

Recent controversy has arisen about the use of the Gustilo and Anderson[11] classification system because of evidence of poor interobserver agreement in classifying fractures by this method. A recent study shows that the agreement on classification of specific fractures is only 60% between different orthopedic surgeons shown the same fractures.[14] Despite disagreement in classifying the fractures, one of the most useful aspects of this system is its correlation with risk of infection and/or other complications. Infection rates for different fracture types have been reported as: type 1, 0% to 2%; type 2, 2% to 5%; type 3A, 5% to 10%; type 3B, 10% to 50%; type 3C, 25% to 50% (**Box 2**).[11,15–17]

INFECTION AND ANTIBIOTIC PROTOCOLS

Infection is the most common morbidity in an open fracture. All open fractures are, by definition, considered contaminated or dirty wounds, and should be managed accordingly.[18] Patzakis and colleagues[19] described antibiotic treatment of open fractures as therapeutic and not prophylactic, because of the high infection rate in this type of injury where antibiotics are not used.

Factors commonly causing increase in infection rates are comminuted fracture patterns, high-velocity injuries, and large amounts of soft tissue loss.[20] Local defenses

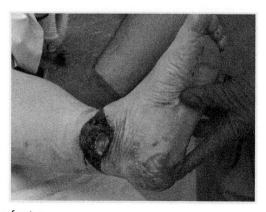

Fig. 1. Type 3 open fracture.

Box 2
Rates of infection in Gustilo and Anderson[11] open fractures

Type I: 0% to 2%

Type II: 2% to 5%

Type IIIA: 5% to 10%

Type IIIB: 10% to 50%

Type IIIC: 25% to 50%

---

in the soft tissue can cope with up to 10^5 organisms per gram of tissue without the development of infection.[21] When more bacteria are present, infection results. Moore and colleagues[22] showed that open fracture bacterial counts greater than 10^5 resulted in infection 50% of the time; with counts less than this, the infection rate decreased to 5%. Injuries with large amount of devitalized tissue require lower levels of bacteria to reach infection. Merritt[23] shows that the bacterial load is imperative to predicting infection rates. He also shows that levels of contamination before debridement do not increase the risk of infection.

Risk of bacterial introduction and compromise to soft tissue structures must be managed properly in the initial evaluation as well as the surgical management of even minor open fractures.[24,25] Some advocate obtaining immediate wound cultures in open fractures; however, this has been shown to be of little use in identifying organisms that contaminate such wounds. It is reported that 92% of open fracture infections were the result of nosocomial bacteria.[1,26] Only about 8% of organisms cultured from initial swabs resulted as the organism causing eventual infections.[27,28] More accurate cultures were obtained after debridement than were obtained on initial evaluation.[8] Therefore, current recommendations do not reflect the use of immediate wound cultures as a routine procedure in managing open fractures.

In the lower extremities, infection in open fractures can have severe consequences. Fifty percent of the most severe open fractures (ie, 3C injuries) require amputation of the extremity because of arterial compromise. In addition to the risk of amputation in type 3C injuries, the rate of sepsis can be from 25% to 50%.[12,13] High infection rates and increased risk of amputation necessitate immediate antibiotic treatment. Since Patzakis and colleagues[19] first reported antibiotic benefits in open fracture treatment (1974), there has been a reduction of infection of up to 59%.[1,19]

Early administration of antibiotics has shown a decrease in the risk of infection. When antibiotic therapy is administered within 3 hours of the initial injury, there is up to a 6-fold decrease in infection rates.[17,29] However, initial antibiotic therapy should be of a short duration. It has been suggested that a 1-day course of antibiotics is as effective as a 5-day course.[30]

Long-term extended-spectrum antibiotics may increase infection by allowing the growth of certain resistant organisms.[31,32] Although the treatment time should be limited, for each surgical debridement following an open fracture, 3 days of antibiotic should be administered.[30] If the wound shows active signs of infection, antibiotic therapy should be initiated and maintained as the patient requires.

Recommendations on specific antibiotic coverage are related to the most common infecting bacteria found in open fractures. The most common are gram-positive cocci and gram-negative bacilli. For type 1 injuries, a first-generation cephalosporin is indicated. Because the most common pathogen isolated from bone is coagulase-positive *Staphylococcus*, cefazolin, which covers this organism, is frequently used. Between 1 and 2 g of intravenous (IV) cefazolin every 8 hours for 24 hours after wound closure is recommended.[1] For type 2 and 3 injuries, an aminoglycoside such as gentamycin or tobramycin is recommended, in addition to the cephalosporin because of the increase in infection by *Pseudomonas* and *Enterobacter* species in type 2 and 3 open fractures.

A common dose is gentamycin, 3 to 5 mg/kg, in divided doses every 8 hours with a 1.7-mg/kg loading dose. If the injury is contaminated by soil or animal feces, it is recommended that penicillin G 10 to 20 million U be given daily, to lower the risk of clostridium infection.[13,17,19] Ciprofloxacin is also considered a viable choice in treating open fractures and bone injuries because of its bone penetration; however, some concern for its inhibition of osteoblast activity and fracture healing is a concern (**Table 1**).[33,34]

During surgery, further antibiotic therapy may be required. This direct local delivery of antibiotics serves to fill voids in bone or tissue. Wounds with large dead space may necessitate the use of polymethyl methacrylate (PMMA) beads. The beads deliver high-dose antibiotic with minimal systemic influence. The beads have been found to release 5% of their antibiotic load in the first 24 hours, which translates to antibiotic levels that are 20 times higher at the site of the wound than with systemic administration. In addition, therapeutic levels have shown up to 5 to 10 days following implantation.[35] Henry and colleagues[36] found a decrease in the level of bacteria as well as a decrease in deep infections of up to 4 times when given with IV antibiotics.

DEBRIDEMENT

Debridement is vital in the treatment of open fracture injuries.[20] All devitalized tissue must be excised, otherwise it can become a nidus for bacterial growth deep in the wound. The primary factor leading to deep infection is improper or insufficient debridement.[12] Any break in the integument causes coagulation by platelets, releasing coagulation factors that cause vasoconstriction, which in turn leads to local hypoxia and acidosis and the eventual recruitment of inflammatory cells. Macrophages then clear debris and stimulate fibroblasts and angiogenesis. For this process to function appropriately, oxygen must be present in the tissues; this is a main pathophysiologic reason for debridement of any and all devitalized tissue following an open fracture–type injury.

When debriding an open fracture wound, care should be taken that neurovascular structures are avoided. Viability of muscle can be evaluated using low-power coagulation stimulation. Nonviable muscle does not contract or twitch with stimulation and should be removed. Scully and colleagues[37] suggest that the viability of muscle can be evaluated by contractility, consistency, bleeding, and color. Healthy muscle bleeds when cut, contracts when stimulated, is firm, and appears pink or red. All nonviable bone fragments should be excised. If left in the wound, nonviable bone can become a nidus for deep infection. Fascia and fat surrounding the wound should be excised because of its avascular nature and susceptibility to infection. The practice of trying

Table 1 Antibiotic treatment of open fractures	
Type of Injury	**Antibiotic**
Type 1	First-generation cephalosporin
Type 2	Cephalosporin plus aminoglycoside
Type 3	Cephalosporin plus aminoglycoside
Suspect clostridium	Ciprofloxacin

to excise as little tissue as possible should be avoided; debridement should be aggressive because of the high risk of infection in open fractures. Open fractures that involve a joint need to undergo a thorough arthrotomy and debridement of the joint as well.[20,38,39]

Typically, more than 1 surgical debridement is necessary for type 3 open fractures, and additional debridement may be necessary to achieve a healthy wound in any type of open fracture. Skin and structures that appear viable with the first debridement may become necrotic and nonviable if circulation is compromised. Adequate daily evaluation and treatment is necessary. A strong predictor of outcome following an open fracture injury is the amount of energy absorbed by the tissue during the trauma. Complicated fracture patterns indicate a higher level of energy transferred to the tissues; days later, necrosis can occur in the soft tissue. Higher energy injuries need multiple reassessments and debridements to stabilize the soft tissues before the fracture can be addressed.[40,41]

IRRIGATION

An important aspect of the surgical debridement is irrigation and flushing of the wound with large volumes of fluids. Irrigation is important to removing any macrocontamination, clotted blood, or loose debris in the wound, which also aids surgical debridement, allowing better visualization of deep level of the wounds and assisting the identification of viable and nonviable tissue. Copious irrigation also decreases the bacterial load of infective organisms present in the wound.[42]

Controversy exists about the choice of both mechanism and solution for the irrigation of open fracture wounds. Some advocate high-pressure pulse lavage, some low-pressure pulse lavage, and others only bulb-directed irrigation. Current data show that a medium-pressure lavage is preferable because of the risk of additional damage to tissue or bone in an already traumatized soft tissue region. Data also show that high-pressure pulse lavage has an increased removal of slime-producing bacteria.[42–44] There is insufficient evidence to make a blanket recommendation, so surgeon choice on a case-by-case basis is currently the standard.

When determining irrigation solutions, some surgeons advocate saline irrigation, some soap irrigation, and others antibiotic irrigation. It has been reported that there is no significant difference between antibiotic irrigation and irrigation with liquid castile soaps relative to infection and bone healing rates in open fractures. However, it is suggested that there is a significant correlation between decreased wound healing with the use of antibiotic irrigation solutions.[42] The mechanical effect of the lavage seems to be more important than the content of the fluid. Type 1 open fractures should receive at least 3 L of pulsed lavage, and type 2 and 3 should receive from 9 L to 11 L.[20]

FIXATION AND STABILITY

Fixation of open fractures is essential, and has multiple benefits for both osseous and soft tissue structures. Stabilization of the fracture(s) can decrease acute complications in injured individuals, such as respiratory distress, shock, and other organ failure. Stabilization also aids in reducing the spread of infectious material, pain reduction, improved wound and soft tissue healing, and better functional outcome.[20,40,41,45] The restoration of length obtained by correct reduction and stabilization is also a beneficial outcome, because it decreases the soft tissue dead space, reducing edema and decreasing infection rates.[23,46]

Multiple methods for stabilizing open fractures are available. The choice should be determined by the judgment of the treating physician. Factors affecting choice of stabilization include mechanism of injury, type and location of injury, soft tissue damage, and overall patient condition.[1] Plaster splint immobilization with k-wires or percutaneous pinning are the conservative options for treatment and have been well documented in the literature. Pinning of open fractures allows for less soft tissue dissection, therefore minimizing soft tissue compromise. Other options include casting, external and internal fixation devices, and traction.

Intra-articular fractures should be fixated at the time of initial debridement. If this is not performed, malunion of the joint surface can result in joint arthritis. Even though fixation should not be placed into a contaminated wound, the benefits outweigh the risks in intra-articular fractures.[47]

External fixation is a common method to treat open fractures. It can be used as temporary fixation for stabilization and it can accommodate the soft tissue compromise associated with a particular wound. It may also allow for distraction of the fracture, which can aid reduction for later implementation of internal fixation devices (**Fig. 2**). External fixation is indicated in open fractures with extensive soft tissue compromise, type 3 injures, and for fixation required immediately in an unstable patient.[1]

Internal fixation is typically recommended for extremity fractures and periarticular fractures. Internal fixation is not indicated in open fractures of the high-energy type or in cases in which the soft tissues covering the internal fixation may be injured.[48,49] In addition, internal fixation should be avoided in comminuted or contaminated wounds. Higher infection rates have been published when using plates for internal fixation in open fractures; however, newer plates and newer application techniques are showing a decrease in these previous reports and studies.[50–52] Infection rates in cases in which internal fixation is used in type 1 injuries are no higher than those reported with closed treatment.[53] When performing internal fixation, incisions should be made straight to the bone, and wide planes of dissection and periosteal stripping should be avoided.[20]

CLOSURE AND GRAFTING

Wound closure is often a difficult factor in treating open fractures. In the past, open fracture wounds have been delayed-closure procedures. This practice is changing,

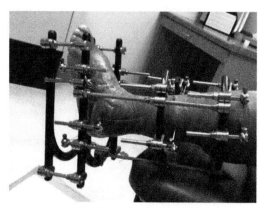

Fig. 2. External fixation device applied to maintain reduction of an open calcaneal fracture.

and current evidence tends toward immediate closure, but there are still conflicting data on the issue. No significant increase in infection rates or delayed bone healing have been found with immediate closure compared with delayed closures.[54] Cullen and colleagues[55] found that most infections are associated with type 3B and 3C fractures of children; subsequently, he recommends that type 3B and 3C wounds should not be closed primarily.[30,55] In addition, if there is any doubt about the contamination of a wound, it should be left open for redebridement, and closure should only be attempted when the wound is clean and edges are viable. Most studies mentioned in the literature regard open tibial fractures. Open tibial fractures have a 10 to 20 times greater risk of infection compared with other bones. Weitz-Marshall and Bosse[56] and Crowly and Kanakaris[57] both suggest the following in deciding whether to delay wound closure:

- Open fractures contaminated with stagnant water or gross contaminants, and farming or boating injuries are not suitable for immediate closure.
- Twelve-hour delay in initial antibiotic therapy, severe comorbidities, and inadequate initial debridement are all contraindications to immediate closure.

Difficulty in obtaining adequate soft tissue coverage is common in traumatic open fracture wounds. Methods to achieve closure include split-thickness and full-thickness skin grafts and the use of muscle flaps. This grafting should be done within the first 3 to 7 days. Grafts or flaps can be placed when the wound is out of the acute inflammatory phase. The use of vacuum therapy in assisted closure of wounds is also a viable method in the management of open fracture wounds. Vacuum-assisted closure (VAC) therapy has been shown to reduce edema, increase local blood flow, enhance granulation of tissue, decrease bacterial load, and accelerate the wound healing process. Wound VACs can be used to aid in both primary and delayed closures.[58,59]

Bone grafting may also be used to fill dead space, or aid in fusion and healing at the fracture site. Bone grafting is not indicated in type 3B and 3C wounds but can be attempted in less severe fracture types. The surgeon must be confident that the wound is free from infection and has an appropriate soft tissue envelope for coverage of the bone graft.[20]

AMPUTATION

In severe open fracture cases, primary amputation must be considered. This decision is based on surgeon preference and experience. Patient tolerance for various treatments of the open fracture must be considered and primary amputation may be the better option for a particular patient, based on the location of the injury and the possible level of amputation. Mangled Extremity Severity Score (MESS) can be used to evaluate lower extremity trauma in severe cases. This system is based on limb ischemia, shock, age, and skeletal or soft tissue injury. In this system, a grade of 7 or more is an indicator for primary amputation (**Table 2**).[60]

In cases in which severe trauma occurs to a digit, with extensive soft tissue loss and neurovascular compromise, primary amputation may be the procedure of choice. The benefit of primary amputation is that these incisions may be closed primarily.

COMPLICATIONS

Complications are common with open fractures, and should be monitored after surgery. The severity of the initial injury is directly related to the incidence of

Table 2
Mangled Extremity Severity Score for evaluation of primary amputation following severe trauma

Consideration for Amputations	Points
Skeletal/soft tissue injury	
Low energy (stab, simple fracture, pistol GSW)	1
Medium energy (open or multiple fractures, dislocation)	2
High energy (high-speed MVA or rifle GSW)	3
Very high energy (high-speed trauma + gross contamination)	4
Limb ischemia	
Pulse reduced or absent but perfusion normal	1[a]
Pulseless; paresthesias, diminished capillary refill	2
Cool, paralyzed, insensate, numb	3[a]
Shock	
Systolic BP always >90 mm Hg	0
Hypotensive transiently	1
Persistent hypotension	2
Age (years)	
<30	0
30–50	1
>50	2

Abbreviations: BP, blood pressure; GSW, gunshot wound; MVA, motor vehicle accident.
  [a] Score doubled for ischemia >6 hours.

complications. Major complications can include soft tissue infections, osteomyelitis, skin compromise, nonunion, delayed union, complex regional pain syndrome, gangrene, and future amputations.

Patients should be monitored closely after treatment of open fractures because of the risk of the significant complications listed earlier. Difficult or poorly healing wounds may need more supervision and management. The need for both clinical and radiographic follow-ups vary in each case.

SUMMARY

Open fractures can be a complicated and challenging injury because of the typical mechanisms of injury, high risk of infection, presence of debris in wounds, difficulty in obtaining reduction/fixation, and need for adequate soft tissue coverage. The combination of both bony fractures and soft tissue damage makes management of open fractures particularly challenging. Any open fracture is considered a surgical emergency that requires appropriate initial and surgical management. Appropriate antibiotic choice should be initiated as soon as possible, preferably within 3 hours of the injury. Surgical debridement and pulse lavage irrigation remains the cornerstone of treatment, with the choice of solution and pressure still being controversial, but with data indicating saline or soap solutions versus antibiotic washes. Stabilization of the fracture as soon as possible aids in decreasing soft tissue damage, edema, pain, and future complications. Wound closure recommendations are trending to early versus delayed closure, but further evidence is required. Adjunct therapies such as the use of antibiotic beads, bone grafts, and wound-VAC therapy may aid in reducing complications and also in the management of open fractures.

REFERENCES

1. Okike K, Bhattacharyya T. Current Concepts review: trends in the management of open fractures. J Bone Joint Surg 2006;88-A:12.
2. Praemer A, Furner S, Rice DP. Musculoskeletal conditions in the US. Park Ridge (IL): American Academy of Orthopaedic Surgeons; 1992.
3. Court-Brown CM, McQueen MM. Management of open fractures. St Louis (MO); London: Mosby; 1996.
4. Court-Brown CM, Rimmer S. The epidemiology of open long bone fractures. Injury 1998;29:529–35.
5. Schaller TM. Open fractures. Available at: www.emedicine.medscape.com/article/1263242-overview. Accessed June 2011.
6. Brenner P, Remmelts S, Marian J, et al. Early soft tissue coverage after complex foot trauma. World J Surg 2001;25(5):603–9.
7. Anderson JT, Gustilo RB. Immediate internal fixation in open fractures. Orthop Clin North Am 1980;11:569.
8. Gustilo RB. Management of open fractures and their complications. Philadelphia: WB Saunders; 1982.
9. Bleck TP. *Clostridium tetani* (tetanus). In: Mandell G, editor. Principles and practice of infectious disease. 6th edition. Philadelphia: Churchill Livingstone; 2005. p. 299–304.
10. Howard F, Duval MK. The complications of surgical wounds. Arch Surg 1960;26:781–2.
11. Gustilo RB, Anderson JT. Prevention of infection in the treatment of one thousand and twenty-five open fractures of long bones. J Bone Joint Surg 1963;52A:453.
12. Gustilo RB. Current Concepts review: the management of open fractures. J Bone Joint Surg 1990;72A:299.
13. Gustilo RB. Use of antimicrobials in the management of open fractures. Arch Surg 1979;114:804.
14. Brumbach RJ, Jones AL. Interobserver agreement in the classification of open fractures of the tibia. The results of a survey of two hundred and forty-five orthopaedic surgeons. J Bone Joint Surg Am 1994;76:1162–6.
15. Gustilo RB, Mendoza RM. Problems in the management of type II open fractures of the tibia. J Trauma 1984;24:742–6.
16. Gustilo RB, Gruninger RP. Classification of type III open fractures relative to treatment and results. Orthopedics 1987;10:1781–8.
17. Patzakis MJ, Wilkins J. Factors influencing infection rate in open fracture wounds. Clin Orthop 1989;243:36–40.
18. Cross WW, Swiontkowski MF. Treatment principles in the management of open fractures. Indian J Orthop 2008;42:377–86.
19. Patzakis MJ, Harvey JP, Ivler D. The role of antibiotics in the management of open fractures. J Bone Joint Surg 1974;56A:532.
20. Gumann G. Fractures of the foot and ankle. Philadelphia: Elsevier Saunders; 2004.

21. Fry DE, Polk HC. Infection in the surgical patient: prevention and treatment. Drug Ther 1982;7:19–28.
22. Moore TJ, Mauncey C, Barron J. The use of quantitative bacterial counts in open fractures. Clin Orthop 1989;248:227–30.
23. Merritt K. Factors increasing the risk of infection in patients with open fractures. J Trauma 1988;28:823–7.
24. Johnson EN, Burns TC. Infectious complications of open type III tibial fractures among combat casualties. Clin Infect Dis 2007;45:409–15.
25. Neubauer T, Bayer GS. Open fractures and infection. Acta Chir Orthop Traumatol Cech 2006;73:301–12.
26. Carsenti-Etesse H. Epidemiology of bacterial infection during management of open leg fractures. Eur J Clin Microbiol Infect Dis 1999;18:315–23.
27. Lee J. Efficacy of cultures in the management of open fractures. Clin Orthop Relat Res 1997;339:71–5.
28. Valenziano CP, Chattar-Cora D. Efficacy of primary wound cultures in long bone open extremity fractures. Arch Orthop Trauma Surg 2002;122:259–61.
29. Patzakis MJ, Wilkins J. Considerations in reducing the infection rate in open tibial fractures. Clin Orthop Relat Res 1983;178:36–41.
30. Dellinger EP, Caplan ES, Weaver LD, et al. Duration of preventative antibiotic administration for open extremities fractures. Arch Surg 1988;123:333–9.
31. Antrum RM, Solomkin JS. A review of antibiotic prophylaxis for open fractures. Orthop Rev 1987;16:81–9.
32. Wilkins J, Patzakis MJ. Choice and duration of antibiotics in open fractures. Orthop Clin North Am 1991;22:433–7.
33. Holtom PD, Pavkovic SA. Inhibitory effects of the quinolone antibiotics. J Orthop Res 2000;18:721–7.
34. Huddleston PM, Steckelberg JM. Ciprofloxacin inhibition of experimental fracture healing. J Bone Joint Surg Am 2000;82:161–73.
35. Henry SL, Seligson D, Mangino P, et al. Antibiotic impregnated beads. Part 1: Bead implantation vs systemic therapy. Orthop Rev 1991;20:242–7.
36. Henry SL, Osterman PAW, Seligson D, et al. The prophylactic use of antibiotic impregnated beads in open fractures. J Trauma 1990;30:1231–8.
37. Scully RE, Artz C, Sako Y. An evaluation of the surgeon's criteria for determining viability of muscle during debridement. Arch Surg 1956;73:1031.
38. Browner BD. Skeletal trauma: basic science, management, and reconstruction. 3rd edition. Philadelphia: Saunders; 2003.
39. Tscherne H, Gotzen L. Fractures with soft tissue injuries. New York: Springer-Verlag; 1984.
40. Chapman MW. The use of immediate internal fixation in open fractures. Orthop Clin North Am 1980;11:579.
41. Chapman MW. Operative orthopedics. Philadelphia: JB Lippincott; 1993.
42. Anglen JO. Comparison of soap and antibiotic solutions for irrigation of lower-limb open fracture wounds. J Bone Joint Surg Am 2005;87:1415–22.
43. Bhandari M, Schemitsch EH. High and low pressure pulsatile lavage of contaminated tibial fractures. J Orthop Trauma 1999;13:526–33.
44. Bhandari M, Thompson K. High and low pressure irrigation in contaminated wounds with exposed bone. Int J Surg Investig 2000;2:179–82.
45. Worlock P, Slack R. The prevention of infection in open fractures: an experimental study of the effect of fracture stability. Injury 1994;25:31–8.
46. Merritt K, Dowd JD. Role of internal fixation in infection of open fractures: studies with *Staphylococcus aureus* and *Proteus mirabilis*. J Orthop Res 1987;5:23–8.

47. Healy KM, Danis KM. Treatment of open fractures. Clin Podiatr Med Surg 1995; 12:4.
48. Sirkin M, Sanders R. A staged protocol for soft tissue management in the treatment of complex pilon fractures. J Orthop Trauma 2004;18:32–8.
49. Watson JT, Moed BR. Treatment protocol based on severity of soft tissue injury. Clin Orthop Relat Res 2000;375:78–90.
50. Clifford RP, Beauchamp CG. Plate fixation of open fractures of the tibia. J Bone Joint Surg Br 1988;70:644–8.
51. Cole PA, Zlowodzki M. Treatment of proximal tibia fractures using the less invasive stabilization system: surgical experience and early clinical results. J Orthop Trauma 2004;18:528–35.
52. Frankhauser F, Gruber G. Minimal-invasive treatment of distal femoral fractures with the LISS (less invasive stabilization system). Acta Orthop Scand 2004;75: 56–60.
53. Rittman WW, Schibli M, Matter P, et al. Open fractures. Long term results in 200 consecutive cases. Clin Orthop 1979;138:132–40.
54. Delong WG, Born CT. Aggressive treatment of 119 open fracture wounds. J Trauma 1999;46:1049–54.
55. Cullen MC, Roy DR, Crawford AH, et al. Open fracture of the tibia in children. J Bone Joint Surg 1996;78:1039–47.
56. Weitz-Marshall AD, Bosse MJ. Timing of closure of open fractures. J Am Acad Orthop Surg 2002;10:379–84.
57. Crowly DJ, Kanakaris NK. Debridement and wound closure of open fractures: the impact of the time factor on infection rates. Injury 2007;38:879–89.
58. Defranzo AJ, Argenta LC. The use of vacuum-assisted closure therapy for the treatment of lower-extremity wounds with exposed bone. Plast Reconstr Surg 2001;108:1184–91.
59. Labler L, Keel M. Vacuum-assisted closure (VAC) for temporary coverage of soft-tissue injury in type III open fracture of the lower extremity. Eur J Trauma 2004;30: 305–12.
60. Gregory RT, Gould RJ, Peclet M, et al. The mangled extremity syndrome (MES): a severity grading system for multisystem injury of the extremity. J Trauma 1985; 25:1147–50.

Treatment of the Neglected Achilles Tendon Rupture

Nicholas J. Bevilacqua, DPM

KEYWORDS

• Achilles • Neglected • Chronic rupture • FHL transfer

Achilles tendon rupture occurs frequently and if not managed appropriately may result in significant disability. Prompt diagnosis of an acute rupture and early initiation of treatment generally lead to optimal results. Acute Achilles tendon ruptures may be missed or misdiagnosed up to 25% of the time[1] or the patient may not seek immediate medical care because they are still able to ambulate and the pain is tolerable. A delay in treatment worsens the outcome and treatment options become more limited. This article focuses on the treatment options for the neglected Achilles tendon rupture.

The Achilles tendon is the largest tendon in the human body. It is made up of a confluence of tendinous contributions from the gastrocnemius and soleus muscles. This complex is known as the triceps surae. The plantaris muscle is also found in the posterior aspect of the leg, originating on the lateral condyle of the femur, and forms a tendon that passes between the gastrocnemius and soleus and runs medial to the Achilles tendon and inserts directly onto the posterior aspect of the calcaneus. The gastrocnemius, the largest of the 3, is composed of a medial and lateral head. The muscle originates on the posterior aspect of the femoral condyle and courses distally to span 3 joints (knee, ankle, and subtalar joint). Therefore, the position of each of these joints influences the tension placed across the gastrocnemius muscle-tendon unit.[2] The fibers of the gastrocnemius form an aponeurosis with the muscle fibers posterior.

The soleus muscle originates from the posterior aspect of the tibia and fibula below the knee and therefore only the ankle and subtalar joint affect the tension across this muscle-tendon unit. The fibers unite to form an aponeurosis with the muscle fibers anterior. The combined aponeuroses of gastrocnemius and soleus converge to form the Achilles tendon, which inserts on the central one-third of the posterior aspect of the calcaneus.

The Achilles tendon is the strongest and thickest tendon in the human body and can be subjected to loads 2 to 3 times the body weight when walking and up to 10 times the body weight with certain athletic activities.[3,4] Most Achilles ruptures are a result of indirect trauma, either by a sudden stretch (eccentric loading) or a forceful contraction

North Jersey Orthopaedic Specialists, 730 Palisade Avenue, Teaneck, NJ 07666, USA
E-mail address: Nicholas.bevilacqua@gmail.com

Clin Podiatr Med Surg 29 (2012) 291–299
doi:10.1016/j.cpm.2012.01.004
0891-8422/12/$ – see front matter © 2012 Elsevier Inc. All rights reserved.

(concentric loading) producing an overload beyond the tensile strength of the tendon. However, spontaneous low-energy ruptures may occur in the presence of underlying Achilles tendinosis.[5]

A rupture may also be associated with systemic disorders (inflammatory conditions, autoimmune disorders, exposure to fluoroquinolone antibiotics, and systemic steroids[6–9]) and local disorders (injectable steroids, collagen abnormalities, and repetitive microtrauma to the tendon[10,11]). Achilles tendinopathy, in particular Achilles tendinosis, results in degeneration within the tendon, which may be a predisposing factor in rupture.

The Achilles tendon is the most injured tendon in the lower extremity. The incidence of Achilles tendon ruptures reportedly occurs in up to 18 of 100,000 people, most often in athletic men in their 20s and 30s.[12]

Most injuries occur during sports-related activities in the recreational athlete, also known as the weekend warrior.[3] Recreational athletes are more prone to ruptures because of their partial sedentary lifestyle combined with intermittent activities. This situation is in contrast to the professional athlete who is consistently exercising, resulting in a thicker stronger tendon.[3,13]

A rupture is considered chronic if treatment is delayed longer than 4 weeks.[14,15] Contraction of the gastrocnemius-soleus complex occurs as early as 3 to 4 days after rupture.[16] Neglected or chronic Achilles tendon rupture is a disabling injury and has the potential to cause significant loss of function.

DIAGNOSIS

An acute Achilles tendon rupture is often diagnosed through patient history. The patient often complains of pain or discomfort on the posterior lower leg along the Achilles tendon. The patient has significant alteration in gait and complains of unsteadiness, and may notice weakness compared with the contralateral limb. The patient finds it difficult going up and down stairs. Close evaluation of the patient's gait often reveals an antalgic gait with loss of push-off strength and limited propulsion.

In most cases, the patient experiences pain, hears an audible pop, and describes being shot or getting hit with a bat in the back of their leg. However, at times, the pain is not severe and the patient is able to ambulate and, as a result, does not seek medical care. It may be weeks or months before the patient is referred or decides to pursue treatment. Continued functional impairment and alterations in gait cause the patient to seek medical attention.

The physical examination may reveal a palpable gap initially, but with delayed presentation, a bulbous segment may be palpated (**Fig. 1**). This bulbous segment represents disorganized, irregular fibrous tissue and, over time, as the calf muscles contract, the fibrous tissue stretches and heals in an elongated position (**Fig. 2**). As a result, a functional deficit is noted because of loss of mechanical efficiency of the triceps surae complex.[17] On examination, there is increased dorsiflexion, with weakened plantarflexory strength compared with the contralateral limb. There is often calf atrophy and inability to perform a single-leg heel raise. Clinical tests may assist in diagnosis. The Thompson test, in which the patient lies prone with feet hanging over the edge of the examination table and the clinician squeezes the calf muscle to stimulate contraction, is a highly predictive and sensitive test for Achilles tendon rupture and is considered positive (rupture) when there is a lack of plantar flexion response when the calf is squeezed.[18] However, in chronic ruptures, this test may not be so reliable. Thompson and Doherty[18] noted that in chronic ruptures the tendon might adhere to surrounding structures, leading to a weak plantar flexion response when the calf is squeezed.

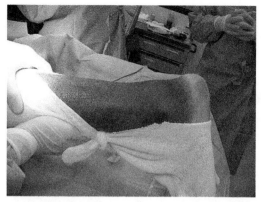

Fig. 1. Bulbous tendon noted in a chronic rupture, representing disorganized, irregular fibrous scar tissue filling in gap.

It is also helpful to examine the resting tension position of the feet with the patient lying prone on the table with the knee flexed at 90°, as described by Matles.[19] Normally, flexing the knee causes the gastrocnemius muscle to shorten, leading to plantar flexion of the foot. With an Achilles tendon rupture, the affected foot often lies in slight dorsiflexion compared with the uninjured side.[3] This test proves valuable in chronic ruptures as well.

Physical examination findings are fairly consistent and are often all that is needed for acute ruptures; however, in the case of a neglected rupture, magnetic resonance imaging (MRI) is helpful in determining the extent of tendon damage and the size of the gap. MRI is an essential component of the surgical plan, because the distance between tendon ends has a direct effect on the surgical decision. MRI allows for a more detailed evaluation of the tendinous structures and determination of the extent of degeneration or scar tissue present (**Fig. 3**).

TREATMENT

Neglected Achilles tendon ruptures are difficult to treat, and surgical reconstruction is superior to conservative care for optimal outcome.[20] Conservative therapy should be

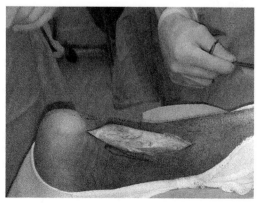

Fig. 2. In chronic ruptures, the Achilles tendon often appears dull, irregular in shape, and is adherent to the surrounding fascia.

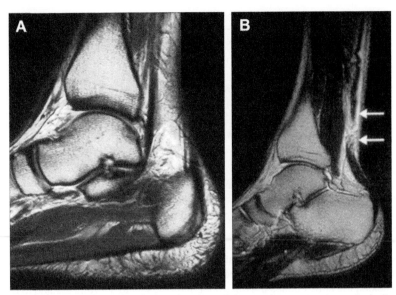

Fig. 3. (*A*) MRI allows for a detailed evaluation of the tendinous structures, including the quality of the flexor halluces longus tendon for potential transfer. (*B*) MRI used for surgical planning to assess the size of the gap between ruptured tendon ends (*arrows*).

reserved for those who are not surgical candidates or those with a sedentary lifestyle who do not have significant functional deficit and are able to perform their activities of daily living.[17] A chronic Achilles rupture results in weakened ankle plantar flexion and abnormal gait. Patients may develop a calcaneal gait, which leads to increased pressure to the plantar heel and may cause significant pain, callus, or ulceration on the heel. In this situation, bracing is used to control ankle motion and to control and accommodate the calcaneal gait. Typical bracing includes ankle foot orthosis, customized boots (Charcot restraint orthotic walker), or a patella tendon-bearing orthosis. Although a brace never restores full function of the leg, it assists in ambulation and improves stability of the lower leg. A structured rehabilitation program should be considered to strengthen the remaining flexor muscles to help compensate for the loss of Achilles function.[17]

Surgical management should be considered for the active individual. The treatment goal is to restore the continuity of the tendon with a length-tension relationship as close to normal as possible. In chronic ruptures, the resultant gap between tendon ends, scarring, and contraction of the gastrocnemius-soleus complex often make end-to-end repair impossible. Porter and colleagues[21] found an average gap of 3 to 5 cm between the tendon ends once the tendon ends were debrided in a series of patients treated 4 to 12 weeks from the time of injury. However, there is considerable variability in the magnitude of the gap between tendon ends.[17]

Numerous techniques have been described for the management of chronic Achilles tendon ruptures. Kuwada[22] and, later, Den Hartog[23] have proposed reported treatment options available to the surgeon depending on the size of the tendon gap after debridement of tendon ends. Smaller gaps (≤2 cm) can often be repaired with an end-to-end technique.[22,23] An end-to-end repair may also be attempted for gaps up to 3 cm. For slightly larger defects (3 cm), tendon mobilization may be performed by placing a Krakow stitch at the proximal segment and applying manual tension for several minutes. However, the surgeon must refrain from repairing the tendon with excessive tension and therefore the surgeon should not hesitate to perform a fascial advancement for gap reduction.[23]

Several fascial advancement options are available, the most common being the gastrocnemius recession, V-Y advancement, and turndown flap.[23] For smaller defects (2–3 cm), a gastrocnemius recession usually permits end-to-end repair. For larger defects (>3 cm), a V-Y advancement or a turndown flap generally allows for direct repair.

A gastrocnemius recession may be performed within the same incision or through a separate incision to reduce the extent of dissection. The gastrocnemius aponeurosis is bluntly separated from the underlying soleus muscle belly. The aponeurosis is then transected. After recession, the proximal tendon segment is manually tensioned and if inadequate lengthening is achieved, a second recession may be performed to the deeper soleus muscle. An end-to-end repair can then be performed using the surgeon's preferred suture technique. Determining appropriate tension is paramount for optimal outcome. The surgeon may use the contralateral ankle as reference.

A gap of 2 to 5 cm between the ruptured tendon ends requires a myotendinous lengthening procedure to bridge the gap. The V-Y myotendinous lengthening procedure was first described by Abraham and Pankovish.[24] These investigators described making an inverted V incision into the tendinous portion of the myotendinous junction, with the arms made approximately 1.5 times the length of the tendon defect; the incision is repaired in a Y fashion. This technique allows the tendon to be advanced, permitting end-to-end repair for defects up to 6 cm, and its use has been reported for defects up to 8 cm.

Advancement of more than 5 cm has been suggested to result in increased muscle weakness. Takao and colleagues[25] reported strength deficits up to 23% on 10 patients treated with gastrocnemius fascial flaps for neglected Achilles ruptures. Us and colleagues[26] noted a reduction in peak torque of up to 23% in patients after a V-Y lengthening alone was performed for a neglected rupture. Therefore, the V-Y advancement should be augmented with a tendon transfer. The surgeon should consider performing a tendon transfer to augment any repair that requires lengthening to achieve an end-to-end repair to add plantarflexion strength.

Tendon transfers have been well described in the literature for chronic ruptures and include using the peroneus brevis, flexor digitorum longus (FDL), and flexor halluces longus (FHL) tendons.[27–30] Mann and colleagues[27] combined an FDL tendon transfer with a fascial turndown in 7 patients, and 6 of these patients had good or excellent results. Den Hartog[23] described an FHL transfer with a gastrocnemius turndown flap. Elias and colleagues[5] described a V-Y Achilles slide enabling end-to-end repair for defects up to 8 cm and augmented the repair with an FHL tendon transfer. These investigators found a 22% loss of plantarflexion strength as well as a 5° loss of active range of motion in 15 consecutive patients treated for defects ranging from 5 cm to 8 cm. American Orthopaedic Foot and Ankle Society (AOFAS) scores were all good to excellent, averaging 94.1/100. Seventy-three percent of the patients were able to perform a single-leg heel raise on the operative limb.

The FHL is an ideal tendon to use and is well suited for tendon transfer to augment neglected Achilles tendon repairs. The FHL tendon offers stronger plantarflexion and the axis of contraction is more in line with the Achilles than the FDL and peroneus brevis tendons.[20] The FHL tendon fires in-phase with the Achilles tendon and maintains normal muscle balance around the ankle. The relative proximity to the Achilles and ease of harvest further support its use, and little functional impairment is noted with harvest.[23] FHL transfer with an interference screw eliminates the need for a separate incision. Herbst and colleagues[31] reported damage to the medial plantar nerve with harvesting the FHL tendon with a 2-incision technique. The added morbidity and increased surgical time make a single-incision approach attractive.

AUTHOR'S PREFERRED APPROACH

After appropriate workup and surgical planning the patients are scheduled for operative management. Most patients receive a regional block of the operative leg preoperatively to assist with perioperative pain control. Patients are then brought into the operating room and placed prone on the operating table. A well-padded thigh tourniquet is applied and used for hemostasis. All extremities are padded appropriately. The operative extremity is prepared and draped in the usual manner.

An incision is made along the posterior medial aspect of the Achilles tendon. The incision begins at the myotendinous juncture and extends distally at the insertion of the tendon on the posterior calcaneus. Placing the incision medially avoids the sural nerve and allows for easier access to the FHL tendon for harvest. The incision is deepened down through the subcutaneous layer, minimizing undermining and using a no-touch technique to the skin edges. The incision is carried down to the paratenon, which is longitudinally incised in the middle of the tendon. There is often proliferation of scar tissue and the gap may be filled in with fibrovascular tissue (see **Fig. 2**). The interposing scar tissue must be resected to the level of normal tendon fibers. This strategy often increases the size of the defect between tendon ends. The surgeon is discouraged from limiting debridement for fear of repair. After necessary debridement, the gap between tendon ends is measured.

With smaller gaps measuring less than 2 cm, an end-to-end approach may be attempted. A Krakow locking stitch using a heavy braided nonabsorbable suture may be placed on the proximal tendon stump and tendon mobilization is performed. The surgeon is cautioned against repairing the tendon with excessive tension and the surgeon should therefore perform a fascial advancement for gap reduction. In cases of neglected Achilles rupture, the average gap between tendon ends is 3 cm to 5 cm.[21] Gaps greater than 3 cm likely require a fascial advancement, and an FHL transfer should be considered with all neglected Achilles repairs requiring fascial advancement.

The FHL tendon is harvested through the same incision and the transfer is secured with an interference screw using a technique described by Elias and colleagues,[5] Den Hartog,[23] and Cottom and colleagues.[32] The posterior fascia is incised longitudinally, exposing the underlying FHL muscle belly. Identification is confirmed with hallux range of motion. The FHL muscle belly is followed distally until the tendon is identified. The tendon is then retracted, with care taken to protect the posterior tibial artery, nerve, and vein. The tendon is then transected as distally as possible, with the ankle and hallux firmly held in maximum plantarflexion. The FHL tendon is mobilized and a whip-stitch is placed at the end of the tendon. The superior aspect of the calcaneal tuberosity is identified and freed of soft tissue. A guidewire for an interference screw is inserted anterior to the Achilles insertion into the superior aspect of the calcaneus and drilled through the calcaneus, exiting the plantar skin (**Fig. 4**). The tendon is measured and the corresponding reamer is used to drill over the guidewire from superior to inferior, with care taken to avoid penetrating the inferior border of the calcaneus. A suture passer is then used to pull the FHL tendon through the bone tunnel. The FHL is pulled to the required tension with the foot held in plantarflexion and the interference screw is inserted. The surgeon may use the contralateral limb as a guide to determine proper foot positioning while tensioning the FHL tendon.

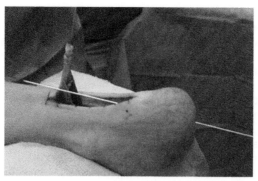

Fig. 4. The FHL tendon is mobilized and a whipstitch is placed at the end of the tendon. A guidewire for an interference screw is inserted through the calcaneus from superior to inferior and exits the plantar skin.

If not already done, a Krakow locking stitch using a heavy, braided, nonabsorbable suture is placed on the proximal tendon stump. The gastrocnemius aponeurosis is exposed proximally in preparation for a V-Y advancement using a technique originally described by Abraham and Pankovish[24] and later Elias and colleagues.[5] An inverted V incision is made through the gastrocnemius aponeurosis, leaving the underlying muscle fibers intact. The apex of the V is placed midline at the proximal aspect of the aponeurosis. The arms extend distally and exit the medial and lateral borders of the tendon. The arms of the V should measure at least 1.5 times the length of the gap. In more extensive gaps (larger than 5 cm) Elias and colleagues[5] recommend extending the length of the limbs to 2 times the measured gap.

A Krakow locking stitch is then placed on the distal stump of the Achilles tendon. Slow, gentle, but consistent traction is applied to the proximal tendon stump, advancing the tendon distally. Traction is continued until an end-to-end repair is possible. It is important to minimize disruption to the underlying muscle fibers and care is taken not to detach the tendon during the slide. The gap is reduced and the end-to-end repair is completed. The proximal site is closed, creating an inverted Y.

Careful layered closure of the peritendinous tissue is performed. The healing potential of the repair is greatly enhanced by preserving the integrity of the peritendinous structures, and adhesions are reduced as well.[2] The wound is dressed and patients are placed in a bulky compressive dressing; a posterior splint is applied in the operating room and removed at 2 weeks. Patients are then placed in an Achilles walking boot with heel lifts, perform protected weight bearing with crutches, and begin an individualized rehabilitation program that includes active plantarflexion and dorsiflexion to neutral. At 4 weeks, patients may bear weight as tolerated in the walking boot. The heel lifts are removed as tolerated, and after 8 weeks, patients may begin to be weaned off the boot. Physical therapy continues to progress range of motion, strength, endurance, and proprioception.

SUMMARY

Neglected Achilles tendon ruptures result in significant functional impairment, and surgery should be considered to restore continuity to the tendon to achieve a near normal length-tension relationship. MRI assists the surgeon in determining the gap between ruptured tendon ends, but it is important to realize that after debridement, the gap often increases. A treatment algorithm guides the surgeon and gives treatment recommendations according to the size of defect.[22]

For smaller defects (up to 2 cm), often an end-to-end repair is possible. The surgeon may manually mobilize the tendon with gentle axial traction applied to the proximal segment to allow for end-to-end repair. The surgeon must refrain from repairing the tendon with excessive tension and should not hesitate to perform a fascial advancement for gap reduction. A gastrocnemius recession may be performed to enable end-to-end repair for small gaps. For larger defects up to 8 cm, a V-Y advancement permits end-to-end repair, and augmentation with an FHL transfer maximizes outcome. Generally, for defects greater than 8 cm, a tendon allograft or synthetic graft may be considered along with an FHL transfer.

Achilles tendon ruptures are best managed acutely. Neglected Achilles tendon ruptures are debilitating injuries, and one must appreciate the increased complexity of the situation. Surgical management is recommended, and only in the poorest surgical candidate is conservative treatment entertained. Numerous treatment algorithms and surgical techniques have been described. A V-Y advancement flap and FHL tendon transfer have been found to be reliable and achieve good clinical outcomes for defects ranging from 2 cm to 8 cm.

REFERENCES

1. Scheller AD, Kasser JR, Quigley TB. Tendon injuries about the ankle. Orthop Clin North Am 1980;11(4):801–11.
2. Schuberth J. Achilles tendon trauma. In: Scurran BL, editor. Foot and ankle trauma. Achilles tendon rupture. New York (NY): Churchill Livingstone; 1996.
3. Thompson J, Baravarian B. Acute and chronic Achilles tendon ruptures in athletes. Clin Podiatr Med Surg 2011;28(1):117–35.
4. Soma CA, Mandelbaum BR. Achilles tendon disorders. Clin Sports Med 1994; 13(4):811–23.
5. Elias I, Besser M, Nazarian LN, et al. Reconstruction for missed or neglected Achilles tendon rupture with V-Y lengthening and flexor hallucis longus tendon transfer through one incision. Foot Ankle Int 2007;28(12):1238–48.
6. Dent CM, Graham GP. Osteogenesis imperfecta and Achilles tendon rupture. Injury 1991;22(3):239–40.
7. Rask MR. Achilles tendon rupture owing to rheumatoid disease. Case report with a nine-year follow-up. JAMA 1978;239(5):435–6.
8. Mahoney PG, James PD, Howell CJ, et al. Spontaneous rupture of the Achilles tendon in a patient with gout. Ann Rheum Dis 1981;40(4):416–8.
9. Haines JF. Bilateral rupture of the Achilles tendon in patients on steroid therapy. Ann Rheum Dis 1983;42(6):652–4.
10. Kleinman M, Gross AE. Achilles tendon rupture following steroid injection. Report of three cases. J Bone Joint Surg Am 1983;65(9):1345–7.
11. Strocchi R, De Pasquale V, Guizzardi S, et al. Human Achilles tendon: morphological and morphometric variations as a function of age. Foot Ankle 1991;12(2):100–4.
12. Gebauer M, Beil FT, Beckmann J, et al. Mechanical evaluation of different techniques for Achilles tendon repair. Arch Orthop Trauma Surg 2007;127(9):795–9.
13. Saltzman CL, Tearse DS. Achilles tendon injuries. J Am Acad Orthop Surg 1998; 6(5):316–25.
14. Jennings AG, Sefton GK. Chronic rupture of tendo Achillis. Long-term results of operative management using polyester tape. J Bone Joint Surg Br 2002;84(3): 361–3.

15. Gabel S, Manoli A 2nd. Neglected rupture of the Achilles tendon. Foot Ankle Int 1994;15(9):512–7.
16. Bosworth DM. Repair of defects in the tendo achillis. J Bone Joint Surg Am 1956; 38(1):111–4.
17. Padanilam TG. Chronic Achilles tendon ruptures. Foot Ankle Clin 2009;14(4): 711–28.
18. Thompson TC, Doherty JH. Spontaneous rupture of tendon of Achilles: a new clinical diagnostic test. J Trauma 1962;2:126–9.
19. Matles AL. Rupture of the tendo Achilles. Another diagnostic sign. Bull Hosp Joint Dis 1975;36(1):48–51.
20. Mahajan RH, Dalal RB. Flexor hallucis longus tendon transfer for reconstruction of chronically ruptured Achilles tendons. J Orthop Surg (Hong Kong) 2009;17(2): 194–8.
21. Porter DA, Mannarino FP, Snead D, et al. Primary repair without augmentation for early neglected Achilles tendon ruptures in the recreational athlete. Foot Ankle Int 1997;18(9):557–64.
22. Kuwada GT. Classification of tendo Achillis rupture with consideration of surgical repair techniques. J Foot Surg 1990;29(4):361–5.
23. Den Hartog BD. Surgical strategies: delayed diagnosis or neglected achilles' tendon ruptures. Foot Ankle Int 2008;29(4):456–63.
24. Abraham E, Pankovich AM. Neglected rupture of the Achilles tendon. Treatment by V-Y tendinous flap. J Bone Joint Surg Am 1975;57(2):253–5.
25. Takao M, Ochi M, Naito K, et al. Repair of neglected Achilles tendon rupture using gastrocnemius fascial flaps. Arch Orthop Trauma Surg 2003;123(9):471–4.
26. Us AK, Bilgin SS, Aydin T, et al. Repair of neglected Achilles tendon ruptures: procedures and functional results. Arch Orthop Trauma Surg 1997;116:408–11.
27. Mann RA, Holmes GB Jr, Seale KS, et al. Chronic rupture of the Achilles tendon: a new technique of repair. J Bone Joint Surg Am 1991;73(2):214–9.
28. Pintore E, Barra V, Pintore R, et al. Peroneus brevis tendon transfer in neglected tears of the Achilles tendon. J Trauma 2001;50(1):71–8.
29. Leslie HD, Edwards WH. Neglected ruptures of the Achilles tendon. Foot Ankle Clin 2005;10(2):357–70.
30. Lin JL. Tendon transfers for Achilles reconstruction. Foot Ankle Clin 2009;14(4): 729–44.
31. Herbst SA, Miller SD. Transection of the medial plantar nerve and hallux cock-up deformity after flexor hallucis longus tendon transfer for Achilles tendinitis: case report. Foot Ankle Int 2006;27(8):639–41.
32. Cottom JM, Hyer CF, Berlet GC, et al. Flexor hallucis tendon transfer with an interference screw for chronic Achilles tendinosis: a report of 62 cases. Foot Ankle Spec 2008;1(5):280–7.

Compartment Syndrome: A Review of the Literature

Michael Murdock, DPM[a], Mica M. Murdoch, DPM[b],*

KEYWORDS

- Compartment syndrome - Lower extremity - Trauma
- Compartmental pressure

Compartment syndrome has been described as an increase in compartment pressure within an osteofascial compartment. It is generally recognized as a complication of crush-type or high-impact injuries to the lower extremities, burns, or even blood dyscrasias.[1,2] The overall incidence of compartment syndrome in the foot associated with crush injuries is 41%. In 2000, McQueen and colleagues[3] found that 69% of 164 diagnosed compartment syndromes were secondary to a fracture, half of which involved the tibia. Myerson and Manoli[1] found that up to 10% of calcaneal fractures develop compartment syndrome.

Compartment syndrome can be difficult to diagnose because of increased edema and pain in most lower extremity injuries; often, the diagnosis must be based on the severity of the injury as well as the clinical examination.[4] It is essential that an immediate diagnosis is made, followed rapidly by proper surgical treatment to prevent further sequelae, such as tissue necrosis, claw toe deformity, functional impairment, cavovarus deformities, neuromuscular injury, or joint contractures.[1,5] The clinical suspicion of compartment syndrome can be further confirmed by the use of portable intracompartmental pressure monitoring devices. Early fasciotomy can prevent long-term nerve, muscle, or tissue injury. It is particularly important to be aware that patients with polytrauma who are hypotensive are at a higher risk to develop compartment syndrome.

Chronic exertional compartment syndrome (CECS) is another subset of compartment syndrome that has been described as a reversible muscle ischemia in an osteofacial compartment secondary to muscular volume increase during exercise.[6] CECS has been defined as preexercise intracompartmental pressures of 15 mm Hg, followed by a 1-minute postexercise pressure reading of more than 30 mm Hg, and a 5-minute postexercise pressure reading of more than 20 mm Hg.[7] These findings, along with clinical symptoms, lead to the diagnosis.

[a] Covenant Medical Center, 3420 West 9th Street, Waterloo, IA 50720, USA
[b] Broadlawns Medical Center, Des Moines, IA 50314, USA
* Corresponding author.
E-mail address: mmurdoch@broadlawns.org

Clin Podiatr Med Surg 29 (2012) 301–310
doi:10.1016/j.cpm.2012.02.001
0891-8422/12/$ – see front matter

In contrast with the acute traumatically induced compartment syndrome, CECS presents with a history of recurrence during activity in younger athletes. CECS has been described as reproducible, and always intensity or time related. Edwards and Myerson[8] assert that the anterior tibial compartment is the most commonly symptomatic compartment at 45%, followed by the deep posterior at 40%, the lateral compartment at 10%, and the superficial posterior at 5%. Women are more predisposed to CECS than men, and surgical correction is less successful in women.[9] Although the presentation of CECS and acute compartment syndrome are different, if CECS is left untreated, it can become an acute presentation and may result in irreversible sequelae.[10]

PATHOPHYSIOLOGY

The result of increased intracompartmental pressure is irreversible myoneural injury within a given compartment.[11] This irreversible damage is secondary to pressure-induced ischemia resulting in tissue death. Muscle and nerve tissue undergo irreversible damage within 12 to 24 hours. Any event that results in hemorrhage or edema, such as surgical procedures, occlusive dressings, fractures, crush injuries, or reperfusion injury, may increase the intracompartmental pressure and decrease the compartmental vascularization.[11] According to the literature, normal resting compartmental pressure is around 6 to 8 mm Hg.[12,13] In a patient with normal vascular tone, vascular perfusion is diminished, if not ceased, at levels equal to or less than diastolic blood pressure; Matsen[14] found that 64 mm Hg in the forearm and 55 mm Hg in the calf significantly impaired vascular perfusion. Surgical fasciotomy is warranted before intracompartmental pressure reaches diastolic blood pressure.[11]

The cause of compartment syndrome has not been agreed on, but the most widely accepted theory is that of venous hypertension. Matsen[14] found that intraluminal pressure in the venous vessels generally exceeded that of the interstitium in a normal compartment. In any acute edematous event, the interstitial pressure becomes greater than that of the venous network and causes collapse. The vascular interstitial gradient loss results in the loss of capillary vascularization. Other theories have been proposed, such as arterial spasm and arteriole collapse secondary to substantially increased intracompartmental pressure, known as critical closing pressure.[15]

The pathophysiology of CECS is not completely understood, but there are theories in the literature. The fascial sheath enclosing the musculature in the lower extremity is inelastic. When skeletal muscle is exerted, it induces an increase in blood flow and edema to the muscle, resulting in hypertrophy. It has been hypothesized that, during eccentric exercise, myofiber damage results in a release of protein-bound ions, which are osmotically active within a given space or compartment. This increase in osmolarity increases the capillary relaxation pressure, resulting in diminished blood flow.[16]

ANATOMY

It was originally thought that there were 4 compartments in the foot: medial, lateral, central, and interosseous. Manoli and Weber[17] corrected this in 1990 by using cadaver dye injection. They found 9 separate compartments: medial, lateral, superficial, adductor, calcaneal, and 4 interosseous compartments (**Figs. 1** and **2**).[17] The flexor hallucis brevis and the abductor hallucis muscles are within the medial compartment. The lateral compartment contains the abductor digiti minimi and the flexor digiti minimi brevis muscles. The superficial compartment houses the flexor digitorum brevis, the 4 lumbricales, and the flexor digitorum longus tendon; it may or may not contain the medial plantar nerve. The adductor compartment only houses the adductor hallucis muscle.

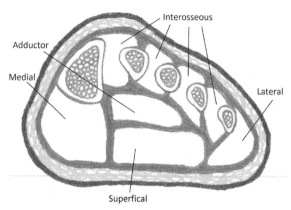

Fig. 1. Cross section of the compartments of the foot.

The quadratus plantae muscle and the neurovascular bundle are found within the calcaneal compartment, including the lateral and sometimes medial plantar nerves.[17] The calcaneal compartment is of utmost importance in assessing a patient for compartment syndrome, because of its small size and numerous neurovascular structures. Because of the large surface area of medullary bone, any traumatic event to the calcaneus predisposes its compartment to increased bleeding and possible intracompartmental pressure increases.[1] The posterior tibial neurovascular bundle enters the foot in the calcaneal compartment but also communicates with the deep posterior compartment of the leg.

The lower leg has 4 major compartments: anterior, lateral, deep posterior, and superficial posterior (**Fig. 3**). The anterior compartment contains the tibialis anterior, extensor digitorum longus, extensor hallucis longus, and the peroneus tertius muscles. It also

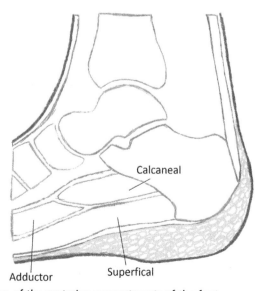

Fig. 2. Cross section of the posterior compartments of the foot.

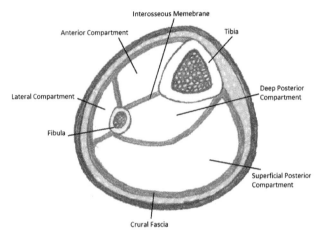

Fig. 3. Cross section of the compartments of the leg.

encloses the deep peroneal nerve and anterior tibial artery. The lateral compartment includes the peroneus longus and brevis muscles, as well as the superficial peroneal nerve. The superficial posterior compartment contains the gastrocnemius and soleus muscles along with the sural nerve. The deep posterior compartment has the tibialis posterior, flexor digitorum longus, and flexor hallucis longus muscles, as well as the posterior tibial neurovascular bundle.

CLINICAL PRESENTATION

Compartment syndrome can be difficult to diagnose. The hallmark presenting symptoms are described as pain out of proportion, parasthesias, poikilothermia (change in temperature), paralysis, and pulselessness.[2] Short of compartment pressure measurements, the most sensitive diagnostic indicator for compartment syndrome is pain on passive muscular stretch within a given compartment.[2] Myerson[18] confirmed this finding. He found that 86% of patients with compartment syndrome had pain with passive, intrinsic muscular range of motion. An adequate vascular examination is necessary to gauge the severity of the patient's symptoms. Often, patients with acute compartment syndrome presentation still have a palpable dorsalis pedis and posterior tibial pulses. It is thought that vascular examinations are not sensitive enough to exclude the diagnosis of a compartment syndrome.

It is also important to assess the patient for any sensory deficits. Two-point discrimination is a better diagnostic indicator for compartment syndrome than pin prick.[18] Because 1 sensory examination may not be enough to rule in or rule out the likelihood of compartment syndrome, serial sensory examinations throughout the clinical evaluation are recommended.

Patients often present in the late stages of the condition when the pain has subsided; this is usually an indication that the muscle tissue is no longer viable. After 6 hours past onset, the prognosis for muscular sparing is poor.[5] For these patients, fasciotomy is not recommended; dialysis to prevent renal damage secondary to rhabdomyolysis is needed.

In contrast with acute compartment syndrome, CECS usually presents as a recurrent cramping, squeezing, or gnawing pain throughout the affected compartment in the lower extremity.[19]

COMPARTMENT CATHETERIZATION

Once clinical suspicion is present, it is essential to have an objective measurement of the severity of the deformity. Compartment pressures may be obtained using local anesthesia. The intracompartmental pressure can be attained by using any of the available commercial pressure devices (Stryker Corp., Digital Quickset, Ace Medical, Pressure Sense Monitor). Fulkerson[11] has some recommendations for appropriate compartmental pressure approaches. Each interosseus compartment can be entered dorsally and the adductor compartment can be measured if the gauge is driven deep through the interosseus compartment. The medial compartment can be accessed approximately 4 cm distal to the medial malleolus. This same approach can be further deepened through the medial intermuscular septa to enter the calcaneal compartment. The superficial compartment is obtained by advancing the gauge into the arch, just deep to the flexor digitorum brevis muscle belly. Inferior to the fifth metatarsal base, the catheter can be inserted to assess the lateral compartment. The anterior, lateral, and superficial compartments of the leg can be entered directly over the compartment (**Fig. 4**). The deep posterior compartment is best entered by passing through the anterior compartment and the interosseous membrane.

SURGICAL TECHNIQUE AND TREATMENT

Many investigators agree that, once a compartment syndrome has been identified, the most widely recommended treatment is surgical fasciotomy.[1,11,14] The fasciotomy can be performed under general or regional anesthesia with the patient in the supine position. Many incision types have been presented, and these are generally specific to the particular compartment. The double dorsal incision approach is used often, in conjunction with the medial approach, and gives access to all the compartments. In this approach, incisions are placed dorsomedial to the second metatarsal, allowing

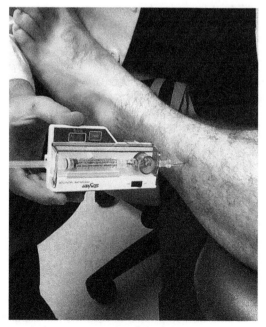

Fig. 4. Measuring an anterior compartment of the leg.

access to the first and second interosseous compartments, and dorsolateral to the fourth metatarsal, allowing access to the third and fourth interosseus compartments. Dorsal incisions are also ideal for repair of any midfoot or forefoot fractures. Depending on which compartments are affected, Myerson[18] also recommends a medial incision to access the calcaneal and medial compartments.[18]

The incision is placed about 4 cm distal to the proximal aspect of the heel, and extends about 6 cm distally, running parallel to the weight-bearing surface. After the soft tissue has been divided, the fascia overlying the abductor hallucis muscle is identified. This fascia is left temporarily intact to allow for plantar dissection to take place. Next, the fascial lining of the abductor hallucis muscle is opened along the length of the incision. The abductor hallucis is then dissected free and retracted dorsally to reveal the intermuscular septa, which form the medial barrier separating the medial from the calcaneal compartment. The septa are then opened using blunt dissection to release the calcaneal compartment. On release of this compartment, there may be some slight herniation of the quadratus plantae muscle belly.[20]

Using the same medial incision, the abductor hallucis muscle fascia is followed plantarly, through the subcutaneous tissue, to reveal the superficial compartment. This compartment is identified and opened to expose the flexor digitorum brevis muscle. With this exposure, the flexor digitorum brevis muscle can be retracted plantarly to reveal the intramuscular septa of the lateral compartment, which are then released.[20] It is generally recommended that the fasciotomies remain open and undergo delayed primary closure 5 to 7 days later (**Fig. 5**).[1,20]

Although the gold standard treatment of acute compartment syndrome is surgical intervention, CECS should be treated initially with conservative measures. Typical musculoskeletal regimes are recommended, such as rest, icing, nonsteroidal antiinflammatory drugs, stretching, strengthening, and orthotic therapy.[6] Surgical intervention is usually reserved for symptoms persisting beyond 6 to 12 weeks of conservative treatment.[21]

There are many different lower leg fasciotomy approaches in the literature. It is thought that the 2-incision, 4-compartment approach, described by Mubarak and Owen,[22] is the most efficient. To allow access to the anterior and lateral compartments, a linear longitudinal incision is placed halfway between the anterior crest of the tibia and fibula, down the leg. This incision placement allows access to both muscle compartments through the intermuscular septum. The second incision is placed posteromedially, about 2 cm posterior to the palpable aspect of the tibia.

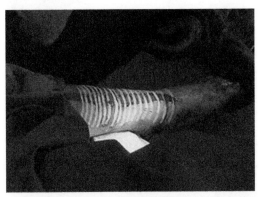

Fig. 5. Open fasciotomy with Steri-Strips used to keep the skin margins approximated in preparation for delayed primary closure.

This incision is generally about 15 cm in length and is linear and longitudinal. Once the posterior superficial compartment is released, the deep compartment can be obtained around the proximal one-third of the tibia and fibula, deep to the soleus muscle. This muscle can be teased away to reveal the deep intermuscular septum, allowing access to the deep posterior compartment.

New literature describes lower extremity fasciotomy using endoscopic assistance and minimally invasive incision placement. In the literature, the procedure is described as a 1-portal endoscopic fasciotomy that is performed by placing a single incision of 2 to 3 cm in the anterolateral lower extremity. The incision is placed 12.5 cm proximal to the lateral malleolus and 5 cm lateral to the tibial crest. The incision is sharply dissected down to the level of the fascia. At that point, the thick fascial septum between each compartment is identified. An incision is placed in the deep fascia of both compartments. Once this incision is placed, a 30° scope is introduced into the fascial incision. A switching stick used to free the subcutaneous tissue from the underlying fascia, and a 30-cm long thoracic straight scissor is used to perform a fasciotomy distally. The arthroscope is slid distally with the scissors to assess the anatomic structures distally.[23]

A 2-incision endoscopic approach has also been proposed. Similar to the previously described technique, 2 incisions are made in the proximal one-third and distal one-third of the anterolateral lower leg. The distal incision is deepened to the level of the deep fascia and the intermuscular septum; a 3-cm transverse incision is made in the deep fascia, thus entering both the anterior and lateral compartments. A large Metzenbaum scissor is then introduced into the distal incision with the arthroscope in the proximal incision, and then fasciotomies are performed in a distal to proximal fashion. Leversedge and colleagues[21] found that 99.8% of anterior compartment, and 96.4% of the lateral compartment, were released with the 2-incision approach.

In 2010, Wittstein and colleagues[24] described an endoscopic fasciotomy of the lower extremity using a 600-mL balloon dissector. A 2-cm transverse incision is placed in the anterolateral aspect of the lower leg between the Gerdy tubercle and the fibular head. The incision is further deepened to the level of the deep fascia. The balloon dissector is then introduced between the superficial and deep fascia. It is inflated with air to create a cavity between the overlying superficial tissues and the myofacial compartment. The balloon is then deflated and removed, leaving a free space that is kept visible with towel clamps. The anterior and lateral compartments are then released, down to the level of the ankle, with endoscopic scissors. Wittstein and colleagues[24] found that 8 of 9 patients were able to return to activity as normal, with no neurovascular insult and minimal hematoma formation.

RECENT CASE STUDIES OF ACUTE COMPARTMENT SYNDROME IN THE LITERATURE

As discussed earlier, the most likely cause of compartment syndrome is secondary to severe trauma. Current literature discusses many instances of compartment syndrome, most of which have atypical causes. It is important to review some of these uncommon cases to promote awareness of the possibility of this pathologic process.

In 2000, Noorpuri and colleagues[25] described a case of compartment syndrome in a rheumatoid patient who underwent revisional forefoot reconstructive surgery. They described symptoms on presentation of an edematous forefoot that was tender to the touch. There were areas of diminished sensation and the patient complained of paresthesias. Although the dorsalis pedis pulse was palpable, they did admit to some capillary refill time delay. The patient also had diminished range of motion to the toes and severe pain on digital extension.[25] The investigators concluded that the ankle block altered the initial presentation of the event. The end result was immediate fasciotomy.

In 2003, Mendelson and colleagues[26] described a case of acute compartment syndrome in a 16-year-old boy after sustaining an inversion injury in a football game. The patient presented to the emergency room that evening with unrelenting pain and his foot in a fixed, inverted position. The patient also had a nonpalpable dorsalis pedis pulse in the affected limb. Compartment pressures were obtained, and the patient had a lateral compartment measurement of 85 mm Hg. Fasciotomy was performed on the lateral aspect of the foot and, on debridement, it was noted that the peroneus longus muscle had torn away from the tendon.

Guo and colleagues[27] described a case of compartment syndrome in a young patient who sustained a supination, external rotation–type ankle fracture in 2010. The patient underwent an open reduction with internal fixation within 24 hours. At 5 hours after surgery, the patient described intractable pain with loss of sensation and parasthesias. The patient's compartments were measured and immediate fasciotomy was performed. Because of the rapid surgical intervention, the patient did not suffer any long-lasting sequelae. Guo and colleagues[27] concluded that a possible cause of the compartment syndrome was a combination of tight skin closure and occlusive dressings. Furthermore, the author offered some recommendations: first, the patient's complaint must be taken seriously; second, physical examination must be carefully performed; and third, do not hesitate to take compartmental pressures.

In 2011, Kemp and colleagues[28] described an acute presentation of compartment syndrome secondary to an ankle sprain. They presented a case of a 24-year-old man who sustained an inversion ankle injury in football. The patient was treated with immobilization and, 3 hours later, the patient presented with extreme pain. The patient's pain was not relieved with opiate analgesics and paresthesias were noted. This patient had an immediate fasciotomy to the anterolateral ankle and, on dissection, the perforating peroneal artery was noted to be actively bleeding. In the current literature, there are multiple cases of compartment syndrome secondary to an inversion injury.[12,13,29–36]

SUMMARY

Compartment syndrome of the foot is a rarely reported complication of lower extremity trauma. However infrequent the presentation, a missed diagnosis can lead to severe and, in some cases, permanent sequelae. Physicians who treat patients with any traumatic injury must be vigilant. Often, classic clinical findings are absent in compartment syndrome of the foot. It is therefore essential to obtain compartmental pressure readings. With early surgical intervention, performed correctly, and proper follow-up care, the pathologic process can be treated without chronic complications.

REFERENCES

1. Myerson M, Manoli A. Compartment syndromes of the foot after calcaneal fractures. Clin Orthop Relat Res 1993;290:142–50.
2. Brey JM, Castro MD. Salvage of compartment syndrome of the leg and foot. Foot Ankle Clin 2008;13:767–72.
3. McQueen MM, Gaston P, Court-Brown CM. Acute compartment syndrome. Who is at Risk? J Bone Joint Surg Br 2000;82:200–3.
4. Ramanujam C. Recurrent acute compartment syndrome of the foot following a calcaneal fracture repair. Clin Podiatr Med Surg 2010;27(3):469–74.
5. Perry M, Manoli A II. Reconstruction of the foot after leg or foot compartment syndrome. Foot Ankle Clin 2006;11:191–201.

6. Wilder R. Overuse injuries: tendinopathies, stress fractures, compartment syndrome, and shin splints. Clin Sports Med 2004;23:55–81.

7. Pedowitz RA, Hargens AR, Mubarak SJ, et al. Modified criteria for the objective diagnosis of chronic compartment syndrome of the leg. Am J Sports Med 1990;18:35–40.

8. Edwards P, Myerson M. Exertional compartment syndrome of the leg: steps for expedient return to activity. Phys Sportsmed 1996;24:31–7.

9. Micheli LJ, Solomon R, Solomon J, et al. Surgical treatment for chronic lower-leg compartment syndrome in young female athletes. Am J Sports Med 1999;27(2): 197–201.

10. Mubarak SJ, Owen CA, Garfin S, et al. Acute exertional superficial posterior compartment syndrome. Am J Sports Med 1978;6(5):287–90.

11. Fulkerson E. Compartment syndrome: a review. Foot Ankle Int 2003;24(2).

12. Botte MJ, Santi MD, Prestianni CA, et al. Ischemic contracture of the foot and ankle: principles of management and prevention. Orthopedics 1996;19(3): 235–44.

13. Dayton P, Goldman FD, Barton E. Compartment pressure in the foot: analysis of normal values and measurement technique. J Am Podiatr Med Assoc 1990;80: 521–5.

14. Matsen FA III. Compartmental syndrome. A unified concept. Clin Orthop 1975; 113:8–14.

15. Burton AC. On the physical equilibrium of small blood vessels. Am J Physiol 1951;164:319.

16. Detmer DE, Sharpe K, Sufit RL, et al. Chronic compartment syndrome: diagnosis, management, and outcomes. Am J Sports Med 1985;13(3):162–70.

17. Manoli A II, Weber TG. Fasciotomy of the foot: an anatomical study with special reference to release of the calcaneal compartment. Foot Ankle 1990;10(5):267–75.

18. Myerson M. Diagnosis and treatment of compartment syndrome of the foot. Orthopedics 1990;13(7):711–7.

19. Glorioso J, Wilckens J. Exertional leg pain. In: O'Connor F, Wilder R, editors. The textbook of running medicine. New York: McGraw-Hill; 2001. p. 181–98.

20. Manoli II A, Dixon D. Compartment releases of the foot. In: The foot and ankle. 2nd edition New York: Lippincott, Williams and Wilkins; 2002. p. 265–78. Chapter 19.

21. Leversedge FJ, Casey PJ, Seiler JG 3rd, et al. Endoscopically assisted fasciotomy: description of technique and in vitro assessment of lower-leg compartment decompression. Am J Sports Med 2002;30(2):272–8.

22. Mubarak S, Owen CA. Compartment syndrome and its relation to the crush syndrome: a spectrum of disease. A review of 11 cases of prolonged limb compression. Clin Orthop Relat Res 1975;81–9.

23. Stein D. One-portal endoscopically assisted fasciotomy for exertional compartment syndrome. Arthroscopy 2005;21(1):108–12.

24. Wittstein J, Moorman CT, Levin LS. Endoscopic compartment release in chronic exertional compartment syndrome. Am J Sports Med 2010;38(8):1661–6.

25. Noorpuri BS, Shahane SA, Getty CJ. Acute compartment syndrome following revisional arthroplasty of the forefoot: the dangers of ankle-block. Foot Ankle Int 2000;21(8):680–2.

26. Mendelson S, Mendelson A, Holmes J. Compartment syndrome after acute rupture of the peroneus longus in a high school football player: a case report. Am J Orthop (Belle Mead NJ) 2003;32(10):510–2.

27. Guo S, Sethi D, Prakash D. Compartment syndrome of the foot secondary to fixation of ankle fracture–a case report. Foot Ankle Surg 2010;16(3):e72–5.

28. Kemp M, Barnes JR, Thorpe PL, et al. Avulsion of the perforating branch of the peroneal artery secondary to an ankle sprain: a cause of acute compartment syndrome in the leg. J Foot Ankle Surg 2011;50:102–3.

29. Ward NJ, Wilde GP, Jackson WF, et al. Compartment syndrome following ankle sprain. J Bone Joint Surg Br 2007;89(7):953–5.

30. Bandy WD, Strong L, Roberts T, et al. False aneurysm: a complication following an inversion ankle sprain: a case report. J Orthop Sports Phys Ther 1996;23(4):272–9.

31. Maguire DW, Huffer MD, Ahlstrand RA, et al. Traumatic aneurysm of the perforating peroneal artery. Arterial bleeding–cause of severe pain following inversion, plantar flexion, ankle sprains. J Bone Joint Surg Am 1972;54(2):409–12.

32. Marks RM, Stroud CC, Walsh D. Pseudoaneurysm of the lateral malleolar artery after ankle sprain: case report and review of the literature. Foot Ankle Int 1999; 20(11):741–3.

33. Rainey RK, Anderson C, Sehorn S, et al. Traumatic false aneurysm of the ankle. A case report. Clin Orthop 1983;176:163–5.

34. Rians CB, Bishop AF, Montgomery CE, et al. False aneurysm of the perforating peroneal artery: a complication of lateral ankle sprain. A case report. J Bone Joint Surg Am 1990;72(5):773–5.

35. Hill CE, Modi CS, Baraza N, et al. Spontaneous compartment syndrome of the foot. J Bone Joint Surg Br 2011;93(9).

36. Myerson MS. Management of compartment syndromes of the foot. Clin Orthop Relat Res 1991;271:239–48.

Puncture Wounds of the Foot

Brent D. Haverstock, DPM

KEYWORDS

• Foot • Puncture • Lower extremity • Trauma

Puncture wounds of the foot, with or without a retained foreign body, are a common presentation to the emergency department, urgent care center, or physician's office. This injury may occur in several settings, ranging from a simple puncture wound occurring at home to a more dramatic work-related injury. The outcome from puncture wounds and retained foreign bodies often depends on the severity of the injury, the penetrating object, and the medical status of the individual who sustains the injury. Most individuals who sustain a puncture wound never seek medical care. They treat the wound at home and are fortunate that complications do not occur. Others may develop an infection or realize that something is wrong with their foot as a result of the injury, such as a tendon laceration resulting in loss of function or a nerve injury rendering an area of the foot numb. Although it is difficult to determine the incidence of pedal puncture wounds, it has been suggested that 10% of such injuries result in a complication.[1] Complications may include a soft tissue infection, deep abscess, osteomyelitis, reactive inflammation, pyogenic granuloma, epidermal inclusion cyst, tendon laceration/dysfunction, and nerve injury.

When an individual presents with a complication related to a puncture wound, the treating physician must carry out a comprehensive history and physical examination and develop an appropriate treatment plan. Delay in treatment may result in significant morbidity or mortality, particularly in the immunocompromised individual (**Fig 1**).

EPIDEMIOLOGY

Pedal puncture wounds can occur in a broad array of circumstances. Most plantar puncture wounds are caused by nails; however, glass, wood, or other metal objects can be the source of the puncture. More than 7% of patients with lower extremity trauma who presented to an emergency department in one survey had plantar puncture wounds.[2] These wounds occurred more often in the months of May to October; however, in the middle of winter in North Dakota, the injury may involve a nail at a construction site, whereas in Florida on the same day, it may be caused by glass on a beach. Superficial wounds generally heal without complications, but deeper

Section of Podiatric Surgery, University of Calgary, Faculty of Medicine, Peter Lougheed Centre, 3500 26 Avenue NE, Calgary, Alberta T1Y 6J4, Canada
E-mail address: brent.haverstock@albertahealthservices.ca

Clin Podiatr Med Surg 29 (2012) 311–322
doi:10.1016/j.cpm.2012.02.002   **podiatric.theclinics.com**
0891-8422/12/$ – see front matter © 2012 Elsevier Inc. All rights reserved.

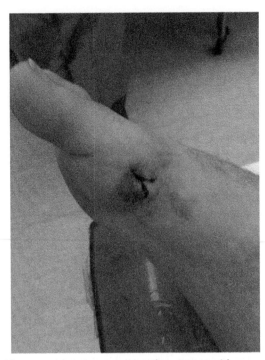

Fig. 1. A 27-year-old man presents to emergency department with a puncture wound to the right foot. The patient was vague as to the nature of the injury.

penetration or a retained foreign body from the puncture is a risk factor for more serious infection. Puncture wounds of the metatarsophalangeal joints or heel and surrounding tissue often penetrate deeper because of the weight-bearing function of these areas of the foot.

The site of the injury on the plantar aspect of the foot has shown variable rates of complications. Patzakis and colleagues[3] evaluated the site of injury on the plantar aspect of the foot to determine variables in complication rates. They divided the foot into 3 zones. Zone 1 extends from the neck of the metatarsals to the end of the toes. Zone 2 includes the area between the distal aspect of the calcaneus to the necks of the metatarsals. Zone 3 is occupied by the calcaneus. In their study, they evaluated the site of injury, condition of the nail, and type of footwear in 36 inpatients and 34 outpatients with nail puncture wounds to the foot. Of the 36 inpatients, 34 (94%) had pyarthrosis, osteomyelitis, or both. Of the 36 inpatients, 35 (97%) had deep puncture wounds in zone 1. In contrast, only 6 of 34 (18%) outpatients had injury to this area. Tennis shoes were shown to predispose to infection with *Pseudomonas aeruginosa*. Based on their findings, they suggested that early hospital admission should be considered for all patients with deep puncture wounds located in zone 1 and for patients who give a history of bone penetration in zone 2 or 3 at the time of injury.

Puncture wounds are common in children who enjoy running around outside unconcerned about the environment they are running in. In a review of 44 children admitted to hospital for puncture wounds of the foot, cultures were positive for osteomyelitis in 7 patients (16%), all involving the forefoot ($P<.04$). The most common pathogen in soft tissue infections was *Staphylococcus aureus*.[4] The most common pathogen in osteomyelitis was *P aeruginosa*. There was no significant difference in the prevalence of osteomyelitis and soft tissue infection based on footwear. There were no cases of osteomyelitis encountered among barefoot children (*P*<.04). In 10 cases (83%), *P aeruginosa* infection (both soft tissue and bone) occurred while the patients were wearing tennis shoes (*P*<.04).

An evaluation of 96 patients who sustained a nail puncture injury of the foot through a rubber-soled shoe showed that 36 (37.5%) were treated conservatively and 60 (62.5%) were treated surgically.[5] Of those treated surgically, 15 (25%) had a foreign body extracted during the procedure. The surgical group had a longer period of time from injury to hospital admission than did the nonsurgical group (5.0 ± 6.8 days vs 2.7 ± 3.8 days, *P*<.05). Treatment success was observed in 91 (94.8%) of the patients, and the median lag time before admission for the less successfully treated group was longer than that for the successfully treated group (10 days vs 2 days, *P*<.002). The less successfully treated group was more likely to receive antibiotics in the community before hospitalization (100.0% vs 47.2%, *P*<.06), and was more likely to be diabetic (40.0% vs 9.9%, *P*<.10).

In a retrospective review of the charts of 80 children admitted to the hospital with plantar punctures, 59 had superficial cellulitis, 11 had retained foreign bodies, and 10 showed osteomyelitis and/or septic arthritis. There was a significant presentation delay in patients from the second and third groups. The most common organisms were *S aureus* or group A *Streptococcus*. Of the 80 children, 34 were treated surgically and 46 were treated with antibiotic therapy alone. All patients with osteomyelitis and septic arthritis were reexamined; at follow-up, all but 1 were asymptomatic apart from residual radiologic sequelae in 4 (**Fig. 2**).[6]

Most of the research to date has centered on puncture wounds of the diabetic foot. Researchers in Montego Bay, Jamaica, performed a study on the natural history of

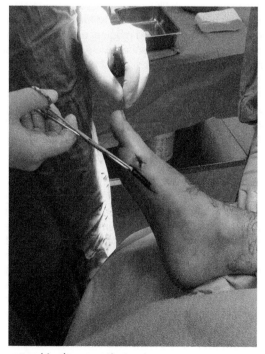

Fig. 2. A pencil is removed in the operating room.

closed pedal puncture wounds in diabetics. A survey was conducted via an interviewer-administered questionnaire on 198 adult diabetics residing in the parish of St. James, Jamaica. The prevalence of a history of at least 1 closed pedal puncture wound since diagnosis of diabetes was 25.8%. Of 77 reported episodes of closed pedal puncture wound among 51 participants, 45.4% healed without medical intervention, 27.3% healed after nonsurgical treatment by a physician, and 27.3% required surgical intervention ranging from debridement to below-knee amputation. The neuropathic foot and the site of the injury (the plantar forefoot) were the variables associated with increased risk of surgical intervention. This study showed that 72.7% of wounds healed either spontaneously or after nonsurgical treatment. This finding means that routine, nonselective surgical intervention for preinfected closed pedal puncture wounds in diabetics is not justified. However, the subset of patients with an anesthetic foot and a wound on the sole of the forefoot should be marked for intensive surveillance and early surgical intervention if infection occurs.[7]

Armstrong and colleagues[8] reviewed the hospital course of 77 diabetic and 69 nondiabetic subjects who had incision, drainage, and exploration of infected puncture wounds of the foot. Diabetics were 5 times more likely to have multiple operations and 46 times more likely to have a lower extremity amputation than nondiabetics. The interval from injury to surgery was significantly longer in diabetics than in nondiabetics. Total lymphocyte count and hemoglobin, hematocrit, and albumin values were significantly lower in diabetics than in nondiabetics. Diabetic amputees had a higher prevalence of nonpalpable pulses, nephropathy, neuropathy, and osteomyelitis compared with diabetic nonamputees.[8]

Lavery and colleagues[9] evaluated the incidence of osteomyelitis in individuals with diabetes who sustained a puncture wound of the foot. The study included 45 men and 21 women who were admitted to the hospital for a foot infection precipitated by a puncture wound. Twenty-two (33%) patients had osteomyelitis based on either a positive bone culture or pathology report. Forty-four patients had soft tissue infections. Patients with osteomyelitis received medical treatment later than patients with soft tissue infections. Significant differences were identified when comparing the time from injury until hospitalization and surgical debridement, and the interval from professional medical evaluation until hospitalization and surgical debridement. The delay in seeking or receiving medical care may dramatically alter the morbidity associated with the puncture wound. Patients with punctures involving the forefoot and patients who wore shoes at the time of the injury were more likely to develop osteomyelitis than patients who had rearfoot injury and patients who were barefoot at the time of injury.[9]

PATIENT PRESENTATION

Most individuals presenting with a puncture wound show a benign looking injury that may be difficult to see. The most common presentation of a puncture wound is a small entry point with irregular skin margins and local ecchymosis. Signs of hemorrhage may also be present. Some may have a more dramatic-appearing injury with a visible foreign object penetrating the foot. Many patients who seek medical care do so because of pain, concerns regarding their tetanus status, or for treatment of a minor soft tissue infection. Patients who have delayed seeking medical care or those with a neuropathic foot often present with a significant wound including local edema and erythema, wound drainage, ascending cellulitis, and lymphadenopathy. The clinical course following the injury may have been uneventful but, in 48 to 72 hours, the picture changes rapidly to the point at which a significant infection is well established (**Fig. 3**).

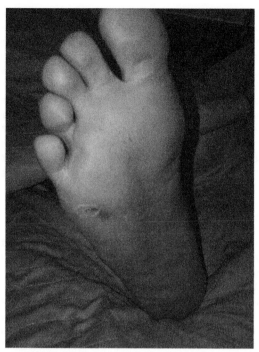

Fig. 3. A 44-year-old man with methicillin-resistant *Staphylococcus aureus* and hepatitis C admitted to hospital with cellulitis of the leg. Examination reveals a puncture wound beneath the fifth metatarsal head.

CLINICAL EVALUATION

When evaluating an individual who presents with a pedal puncture wound, it is important to complete a thorough history before evaluating the foot. It is important to obtain the following information:

(1) When the injury occurred; has it been just a few hours or have a couple of days passed since the puncture wound occurred?
(2) Was the individual wearing any form of footwear at the time of the injury and what was the environment in which the injury occurred?
(3) Did the individual see what the penetrating object was and did they remove any object? If so, did they remove it in toto and do they have it with them?

It is imperative to update the patient's tetanus status to establish whether the individual received vaccination with tetanus toxoid and when they received their last booster vaccine.

When evaluating the foot following a puncture wound, the examiner must first carry out a vascular and neurologic examination. Palpation of the dorsalis pedis and posterior tibial arteries provides a baseline as to the patient's vascular status. If the pulses are nonpalpable, then a vascular consultation will be needed if there is serious infection and surgical intervention is considered. Patients with compromised circulation also require a vascular consultation, even if surgery is not considered necessary. A neurologic evaluation helps to determine whether there is a nerve injury from the penetrating object. Loss of sensation distal to the injury site is a sign that a nerve has been damaged by the object. If it seems that a large nerve is involved, rendering a substantial portion of the foot insensate, microsurgical nerve repair should be performed. This condition must be differentiated from the insensate foot in a patient with diabetic neuropathy. The digits are assessed for mobility to determine whether a tendon laceration has occurred. Careful attention is needed to differentiate the long flexor tendons from the intrinsic flexors of the foot.

The entry site of the puncture is then evaluated. The margins of the skin are assessed for the appearance of jagged or smooth skin edges. The site is inspected for any signs of a retained foreign body. The margins of the wound are gently palpated to again determine whether a retained foreign body is present. The wound is inspected for drainage, malodor, localized erythema, edema, and ascending cellulitis. Crepitus on palpation of the soft tissue may indicate a deep infection with abscess or subcutaneous gas.

DIAGNOSTIC IMAGING

The first step is to obtain plain film radiographs of the foot (**Fig 4**). Metal objects such as pins and nails are easily visible. Glass may be visible if it contains lead or if the fragment is large enough, as will wood splinters that are large enough to cast a shadow on the radiograph. Plastic is not seen (**Figs. 5** and **6**).

Radiographs in the patient with diabetes who has sustained a puncture wound are important to assist in determining whether there is any septic sequelae of the puncture wound.[10] As discussed earlier, patients with diabetes frequently delay seeking medical care. The sepsis that occurs from puncture wounds is often deep to the deep fascia and, because the sole of the foot has thick skin and subcutaneous fibrous septae, crepitus is not as easily appreciated as at other sites. Also, the erythema of the inflammatory response is often minimal in subfascial sepsis. Plain film radiographs may show deep infection, a retained foreign body, or osteomyelitis.

If the patient indicated during the history that the object was thought to be something that is not seen on a radiograph or they are not sure what caused the puncture wound, then further imaging studies are required. Ultrasound is an accurate test for detection of foreign bodies and to assess potential complications such as tendon laceration.[11,12]

Researchers compared the sensitivity for detecting foreign bodies among conventional plain radiography, computed tomography (CT), and ultrasonography in in-vitro models. Seven different materials were selected as foreign bodies, with dimensions

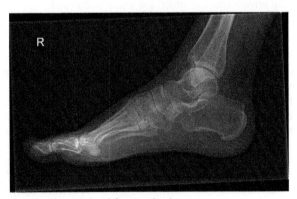

Fig. 4. Radiographs reveal a retained foreign body.

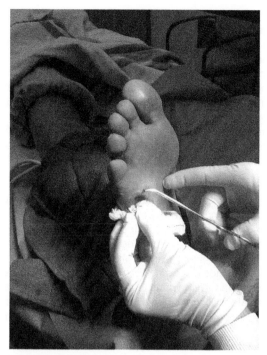

Fig. 5. The foreign body is removed.

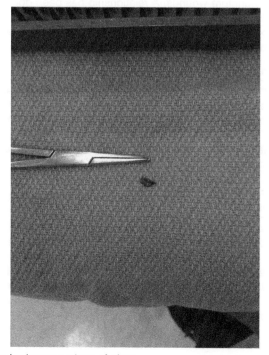

Fig. 6. The foreign body was a piece of glass.

of approximately 1 by 1 by 0.1 cm. These materials were metal, glass, wood, stone, acrylic, graphite, and Bakelite. These foreign bodies were placed into a sheep's head between the corpus mandible and a muscle in the tongue, and in the maxillary sinus. Conventional plain radiography, CT, and ultrasonography imaging methods were compared to investigate their sensitivity for detecting these foreign bodies. It was determined that metal, glass, and stone can be detected with all the visualization techniques used in the study in all of the zones. In contrast, foreign bodies with low radiopacity that could be detected in air with CT became less visible or almost invisible in muscle tissue and between bone and muscle tissue. The performance of ultrasonography for visualizing foreign bodies with low radiopacity is better than CT.[13]

WOUND MICROBIOLOGY

Numerous studies have described the bacterial cause of infections following puncture wounds of the foot. The most common gram-positive organisms isolated in these wounds are *S aureus*, α-hemolytic streptococci and *Staphylococcus epidermidis*. Gram-negative organisms isolated from these wounds have included *Escherichia coli*, *Proteus*, and *Klebsiella* species.[2,4,8,9] Miscellaneous organisms have been isolated from puncture wounds occurring in brackish water. Brackish water is water that has more salinity than fresh water, but not as much as seawater. It may result from mixing of seawater with fresh water, as in estuaries. Organisms isolated from wounds occurring in such an environment include *Aeromonas hydrophila* and *Mycobacterium marinum*.[14]

Pseudomonas infection is a concern in puncture wounds of the foot. *P aeruginosa* is a common gram-negative, aerobic, rod-shaped bacterium that is found in soil, water, and skin flora. *Pseudomonas* is the most common organism responsible for osteomyelitis secondary to puncture wounds. A relationship has been documented between rubber-soled shoes and pseudomonal osteomyelitis.[1,15,16] When a nail or other object penetrates the shoe and then the foot, it inoculates the puncture wound with the pseudomonal organisms found on the shoe.

Management of Puncture Wounds

The management of puncture wounds requires a high level of clinical suspicion because the appearance of these wounds is often benign. The wound should not be dismissed as insignificant. A delay in providing adequate treatment is a factor in the development of complications following a puncture wound of the foot. The approach to managing these wounds depends on whether or not the presenting wound is infected.

MANAGEMENT OF UNINFECTED WOUNDS
Tetanus Immunization

Tetanus is a medical condition characterized by a prolonged contraction of skeletal muscle fibers. The primary symptoms are caused by tetanospasmin, a neurotoxin produced by the gram-positive, rod-shaped, obligate anaerobic bacterium, *Clostridium tetani*. Infection generally occurs through wound contamination and often involves a cut or deep puncture wound. As the infection progresses, muscle spasms develop in the jaw, hence the term lockjaw. Infection is preventable with proper immunization and by postexposure prophylaxis.[17]

Tetanus can be prevented by vaccination with tetanus toxoid. The US Centers for Disease Control and Prevention recommend that adults receive a booster vaccine every 10 years. If patients presenting with pedal puncture wounds cannot recall when they last received a booster, one should be administered.[18] In children less than 7 years of age, the tetanus vaccine is often administered as a combined vaccine that also includes vaccines against diphtheria and pertussis (DPT [diphtheria-pertussis-tetanus]/DTaP [diphtheria-tetanus–acellular pertussis]). For adults and children more than 7 years of age, the Td (tetanus and diphtheria) or Tdap (tetanus, diphtheria, and acellular pertussis) vaccines are commonly used.[19]

Wound Care

In patients who present for medical treatment within 6 hours of the injury and have a superficial puncture wound with no evidence of a retained foreign body, the wound can be probed gently and irrigated with normal saline solution. Jagged or irregular skin edges must be excised. If necessary, this can all be performed under a local infiltrative block. The wound is covered with a sterile dressing that is changed every 6 hours for the first 48 hours, watching for signs of infection. After 48 hours, the dressing is changed daily until the wound is healed.

When a patient has delayed seeking medical treatment or the wound has sustained a deep penetrating injury with significant clinical contamination present, incision and drainage with exploration and irrigation is required. Under a local infiltrative and a regional foot block, the foot is cleansed and prepped. An ankle pneumatic tourniquet is used. The wound must be aggressively debrided of all necrotic and nonviable soft tissue while sharply incising jagged skin edges to decrease the chance of skin necrosis. A deep soft tissue culture is taken. The wound is partially closed over a Penrose drain. A sterile dressing is applied and the patient is instructed to maintain non–weight bearing with crutches until instructed otherwise. The dressing is changed at 48 hours and the wound evaluated. At this time, the drain is removed. The patient is instructed to maintain non–weight bearing until the wound has healed and ambulation can be performed without any pain.

Foreign Body Removal

If the puncture wound has a retained foreign body, consideration must be given to removal of the object. If the object, such as a needle, nail, or gravel, is superficial, removal is simple. The same steps as described for management of a delayed or contaminated wound should be performed along with removal of the object.

A deeper retained foreign body requires intervention under general or spinal anesthesia. A thigh tourniquet allows easier manipulation of the extremity when using diagnostic imaging such as fluoroscopy. When using fluoroscopy, triangulation is often useful in determining the location of the object. Real-time, live imaging is also used as the surgeon attempts to grasp the object. In cases in which the foreign body is not radiopaque, intraoperative ultrasound is helpful in locating and retrieving the object. Irrigation may also flush the object loose from the surrounding tissue.

Antibiotic Prophylaxis

Superficial puncture wounds without clinical contamination or necrotic tissue can be managed without prophylactic antibiotic coverage. The wound is evaluated every 6 hours for the first 48 hours and, if any signs of infection develop, antibiotics should be started.

In deeper wounds with delayed presentation and presence of contamination and necrotic tissue, antibiotics should be started once the wound has been managed and cultures taken. If the patient has an intravenous site, the first dose can be administered via this route. A broad-spectrum antibiotic for coverage of gram-positive and gram-negative organisms and P aeruginosa should be used. Oral ciprofloxacin 500 mg twice daily or levofloxacin 500 mg daily should be prescribed for a 10-day course. If the patient has an allergy or cannot tolerate either of these drugs and there is strong concern for the development of infection, then antipseudomonal penicillin or aminoglycoside may be considered. This requires outpatient intravenous therapy for a few days until the physician is satisfied that a clinical infection has not developed.

MANAGEMENT OF INFECTED WOUNDS

All patients who present with a foot infection secondary to a puncture wound must be considered a medical emergency. As described earlier, a comprehensive history and physical examination must be performed. Baseline laboratory tests, such a complete blood count, erythrocyte sedimentation rate, and C-reactive protein should be completed. Plain film radiographs should be obtained. The patient is taken to the operating room where, under general or spinal anesthesia and with a thigh tourniquet, an incision and drainage procedure is performed. All necrotic tissue is sharply excised and the wound thoroughly evaluated for a retained foreign body. One author advocates creating a small dorsal skin incision, converting a deep track into a tunnel through which irrigation and curettage can be completed. With irrigation of the wound, a foreign body may be removed.[20] Once the wound has been adequately explored, debrided, and irrigated, deep soft tissue cultures are obtained. If preoperative radiographs raise suspicion of an osseous infection, a bone culture should be obtained. The decision to violate the bone should be based on the length of time the infection has been present and radiographic signs of infection such as periostitis, osseous destruction, or lucency. If unsure, further diagnostic tests can be performed following the initial surgical incision and drainage. The wound is lightly packed open and the packing changed every 12 hours. If osteomyelitis is suspected but bone cultures were not taken during the initial procedure, a 3-phase bone scan is completed. If this is negative, then the soft tissue infection only needs to be managed. If the 3-phase bone scan is positive, the next step is to order a white cell labeled bone scan. Again, if this is negative, the soft tissue infection only needs to be managed. If the white cell bone scan is positive, a bone culture can be taken at the time of the secondary debridement and closure. Initially, the patient is started on the appropriate broad-spectrum antibiotics, which are narrowed as culture results become available. Antipseudomonal penicillins, ticarcillin and piperacillin (200–300 mg/kg/d in divided doses, every 4–6 hours), provide excellent gram-positive and gram-negative organism coverage. Third-generation cephalosporins, ceftazidime (1 g intravenously [IV] every 8–12 hours) and cefoperazone (1–2 g IV every 12 hours), also provide Pseudomonas, gram-positive, and gram-negative coverage. Aminoglycosides also provide Pseudomonas coverage and are an option for patients with a penicillin allergy. In adults, intravenous gentamicin is started at 2 mg/kg followed by 3 to 5 mg/kg/d in divided doses every 8 hours. In children, the dosing of gentamicin is 1 to 3 mg/kg/d every 8 hours. All antibiotics must be appropriately monitored and dosed for renal disease and potential toxicity.

Once the infection starts to respond to local wound care and antibiotic therapy, planning for a secondary procedure begins. Between 5 and 7 days should be allowed for the initial infection to respond to antibiotic therapy before performing a delayed primary closure. If a resistant strain of microorganism is isolated, this secondary procedure may be delayed. If it seems that the skin margins will not reapproximate, the use of negative-pressure wound therapy may be considered. The patient is taken back to the operating room for debridement of necrotic or nonviable tissue, wound irrigation, and repeat deep tissue cultures. The wound is closed over a Penrose or closed suction drain.

The foot is evaluated the next day and the drain is removed once the wound site has stopped draining. Antibiotic therapy is based on the final culture results. If the bone cultures are positive, the patient should receive 6 weeks of intravenous antibiotics followed by 4 weeks of oral antibiotics. If the infection only involves the soft tissue, the patient should receive 2 weeks of intravenous antibiotics followed by 2 weeks of oral antibiotics. Inflammatory markers, including the erythrocyte sedimentation rate and C-reactive protein, should be evaluated every few weeks to evaluate the therapeutic process. The patient should be non–weight bearing with a protective cast boot for 2 to 3 weeks until the sutures are removed, and then allowed to bear weight as tolerated in the cast boot until such time that full weight bearing can resume. Physiotherapy or occupational rehabilitation may be initiated to regain strength lost during the period of treatment and recovery from the wound.

SUMMARY

Puncture wounds often appear benign but can go on to cause significant pedal morbidity. Podiatric physicians who treat such wounds should educate local emergency room, urgent care center, and primary care physicians as to the potential complications associated with puncture wounds. Timely referral, recognition of the potential complications, and appropriate treatment ensure that the wound does not advance beyond a puncture wound. If complications have developed, aggressive treatment is required to eradicate the infection and prevent pedal amputation.

REFERENCES

1. Chusid MJ, Jacobs WM, Sty JR. Pseudomonas arthritis following puncture wounds of the foot. J Pediatr 1979;94:429–31.
2. Reinherz RP, Hong DT, Tisa LM, et al. Management of puncture wounds in the foot. J Foot Surg 1985;24:288–92.
3. Patzakis MJ, Wilkins J, Brien WW, et al. Wound site as a predictor of complications following deep nail punctures to the foot. West J Med 1989;150(5):545–7.
4. Laughlin TJ, Armstrong DG, Caporusso J, et al. Soft tissue and bone infections from puncture wounds in children. West J Med 1997;166(2):126–8.
5. Rubin G, Chezar A, Raz R, et al. Nail puncture wound through a rubber-soled shoe: a retrospective study of 96 adult patients. J Foot Ankle Surg 2010;49(5): 421–5.
6. Eidelman M, Bialik V, Miller Y, et al. Plantar puncture wounds in children: analysis of 80 hospitalized patients and late sequelae. Isr Med Assoc J 2003;5(4):268–71.
7. East JM, Yeates CB, Robinson HP. The natural history of pedal puncture wounds in diabetics: a cross-sectional survey. BMC Surg 2011;11:27.
8. Armstrong DG, Lavery LA, Quebedeaux TL, et al. Surgical morbidity and the risk of amputation due to infected puncture wounds in diabetic versus nondiabetic adults. J Am Podiatr Med Assoc 1997;87(7):321–6.
9. Lavery LA, Harkless LB, Ashry HR, et al. Infected puncture wounds in adults with diabetes: risk factors for osteomyelitis. J Foot Ankle Surg 1994;33(6):561–6.
10. Naraynsingh V, Maharaj R, Dan D, et al. Puncture wounds in the diabetic foot: importance of X-ray in diagnosis. Int J Low Extrem Wounds 2011;10(2):98–100.
11. Vargas B, Wildhaber B, La Scala G. Late migration of a foreign body in the foot 5 years after initial trauma. Pediatr Emerg Care 2011;27(6):535–6.
12. Imoisili MA, Bonwit AM, Bulas DI. Toothpick puncture injuries of the foot in children. Pediatr Infect Dis J 2004;23(1):80–2.

13. Aras MH, Miloglu O, Barutcugil C, et al. Comparison of the sensitivity for detecting foreign bodies among conventional plain radiography, computed tomography and ultrasonography. Dentomaxillofac Radiol 2010;39(2):72–8.

14. Chachad S, Kamat D. Management of plantar puncture wounds in children. Clin Pediatr 2004;43(3):213–6.

15. Rahn KA, Jacobson FS. Pseudomonas osteomyelitis of the metatarsal sesamoid bones. Am J Orthop 1997;26(5):365–7.

16. Niall DM, Murphy PG, Fogarty EE, et al. Puncture wound related pseudomonas infections of the foot in children. Ir J Med Sci 1997;166(2):98–101.

17. Otero-Maldonado M, Bosques-Rosado M, Soto-Malavé R, et al. Tetanus is still present in the 21st century: case report and review of literature. Bol Asoc Med P R 2011;103(2):41–7.

18. Hopkins A, Lahiri T, Salerno R, et al. Diphtheria, tetanus, and pertussis: recommendations for vaccine use and other preventive measures. Recommendations of the Immunization Practices Advisory committee (ACIP). MMWR Recomm Rep 1991;40(RR–10):1–28.

19. Vaughn JA, Miller RA. Update on immunizations in adults. Am Fam Physician 2011;84(9):1015–20.

20. Chaarani MW. A new management strategy for puncture wounds of the foot. A case report. Foot 2010;20(2–3):75–7.

Current Concepts and Techniques
in Foot and Ankle Surgery

Versatility of Intrinsic Muscle Flaps for the Diabetic Charcot Foot

Crystal L. Ramanujam, DPM, MSc, Thomas Zgonis, DPM*

KEYWORDS
- Charcot foot • Wounds • External fixation • Muscle flaps
- Surgery • Diabetes

For diabetic foot and ankle wounds, the abductor hallucis, flexor digitorum brevis (FDB), abductor digiti minimi, and the extensor digitorum brevis muscles have most commonly been reported.[1] These flaps allow for low donor site morbidity and decreased functional sacrifice when appropriately used. Intrinsic muscle flaps provide well-vascularized tissue with adequate composition capable of not only filling the defect but also having the ability to withstand high impact forces of ambulation. A case report is presented illustrating successful use of the FDB muscle flap for coverage of a plantar wound resulting from infection in a diabetic Charcot foot.

CASE REPORT

A 55-year-old man presented to the emergency department with a history of a right foot plantar wound infection. Wound duration was approximately 4 weeks with recent onset of increased drainage, foot pain, and subjective fevers. The patient's past medical history was significant for uncontrolled diabetes, peripheral neuropathy, hypertension, and nonobstructive coronary artery disease. He had history of cardiac catheterization without anesthesia complications and admitted recent cessation of smoking and alcohol after a 30-year history of prior use.

Clinical examination revealed an alert and oriented but febrile patient. The foot demonstrated palpable pedal pulses and significant loss of protective sensation. A 3 cm × 5 cm full-thickness wound was visualized at the plantar central midfoot/hindfoot region with exposed tendon and fibrinous base. There was direct probing to bone, purulence at the central aspect of the wound, and peri-wound nonblanching erythema. Radiographic examination confirmed midfoot collapse with osseous disorganization but without a rocker bottom deformity, subluxation, and cystic changes

Division of Podiatric Medicine and Surgery, Department of Orthopaedic Surgery, The University of Texas Health Science Center at San Antonio, 7703 Floyd Curl Drive–MSC 7776, San Antonio, TX 78229, USA
* Corresponding author.
E-mail address: zgonis@uthscsa.edu

Clin Podiatr Med Surg 29 (2012) 323–326
doi:10.1016/j.cpm.2012.02.003
0891-8422/12/$ – see front matter © 2012 Elsevier Inc. All rights reserved.

indicating Charcot neuroarthropathy without definite signs of osteomyelitis. Leukocytosis and hyperglycemia were found on laboratory analysis. Following hospital admission, medical optimization with initiation of empiric broad-spectrum parenteral antibiotic therapy, and vascular work-up demonstrating no arterial occlusive disease in the right lower extremity, the patient underwent staged surgical debridements. Once the acute infection had been addressed, the patient was discharged with an 8-week course of culture-specific intravenous antibiotics.

He was followed in the outpatient clinical setting for local wound care and offloading. Further studies including computed tomography and magnetic resonance imaging confirmed the clinical evidence of prominent plantar cuboid exostosis. Based on the nonhealing wound and imaging findings, he was admitted to the hospital for further staged reconstruction. Ultimately, the patient underwent partial cuboid excision, FDB muscle flap with a biologic matrix dressing, and off-loading with stabilization of the foot and lower extremity with circular external fixation. Biweekly clinic visits thereafter included wire and flap site care with serial radiographs. Six weeks later, the circular external fixation system was removed, and the residual wound was surgically addressed with the use of an autogenous split-thickness skin graft. Further immobilization via posterior splint and continued clinic visits followed until complete healing was observed. The patient was then transitioned to a surgical boot for progressive ambulation and subsequently fitted for extradepth shoes with customized multidensity inlays (**Fig. 1**).

DISCUSSION

One of the first muscle flaps documented in history was in 1906 describing the use of the pectoralis minor muscle for breast reconstruction; however, the first record of pedicled muscle flaps in the lower extremity was introduced in post-traumatic wounds and stasis ulcerations in the 1960s by Ger.[2] Historically speaking, advances in anesthesia, antibiotics, and wound healing gradually popularized the use of these flaps with increasing postoperative success.

Muscle flaps offer unique advantages over other closure techniques when addressing weight bearing soft tissue deficits with bone and joint exposure. They provide durable tissue consistency and longevity for plantar wounds that skin grafts and local skin flaps generally lack. Intrinsic muscle foot flaps for diabetic foot wounds have entertained increasing popularity versus free flaps in diabetic patients based on their relative ease of surgical technique, low donor site morbidity, and quicker operating times.[1] Muscle flaps have also been reported useful in wounds with low-grade infection based on their enhanced vascular perfusion and bacterial clearance.[3] Furthermore, in wounds with significant soft tissue and bone loss, muscle flaps in combination with antibiotic-loaded cement beads or spacers can allow for further staged reconstruction using bone graft.

Much of the existing literature regarding the FDB muscle flap involves soft tissue defects left following resection of tumors, yet its use in the treatment of diabetic foot wounds has gained more attention in recent years based on the increasing prevalence of diabetic foot complications.[4–7] The FDB muscle flap is specifically optimal for foot wounds located plantar centrally or at the heel. The reach of this flap may also allow for coverage of distal lateral defects.[5] The bulk of this muscle varies yet is surprisingly adequate for filling defects extending to bone or joint and provides a durable surface for weight bearing. Dissection of the FDB flap also allows easy access and visualization of associated osseous deformities that may require concomitant correction as seen in midfoot Charcot neuroarthropathy.[7]

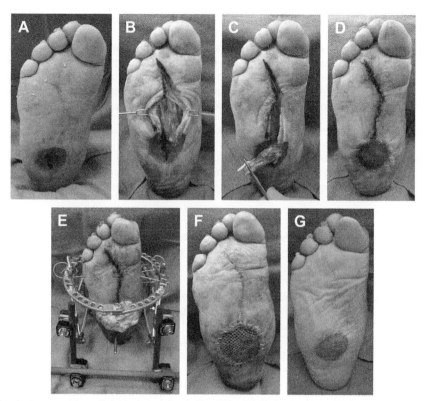

Fig. 1. Preoperative clinical view (*A*) of the diabetic Charcot plantar wound after serial surgical debridements. Intraoperative view (*B*) demonstrating the incision placement for the FDB muscle harvesting and insetting to the recipient area (*C*). Note that a plantar cuboid exostectomy was initially performed through a direct approach of the plantar wound along with percutaneous skeletal fixation of the subtalar and ankle joints. The use of a biologic matrix was initially used to cover the harvested FDB muscle at the recipient site (*D*). Surgical off-loading was achieved with the use of a modified external fixator that also provided stabilization to the foot and lower extremity (*E*). The external fixator was removed at approximately 6 weeks; a split thickness skin graft was also used for definitive closure over the harvested FDB muscle (*F*). Final clinical outcome at approximately 4 months post-operatively (*G*).

Preoperatively, thorough clinical assessment should ensure a wound that is free of acute infection or vascular compromise. The specific type of muscle flap to use is guided by the recipient wound location and proximity to a viable muscle source. Size and muscle bulk should be examined so as to avoid use of inadequate tissues. Meticulous surgical dissection of the muscle flap is performed in a distal-to-proximal fashion, facilitated by use of loupe magnification and Doppler examination to isolate the dominant proximal pedicle and distal minor pedicles. Donor sites for most muscle flaps in the foot and ankle are usually closed primarily. Limitations of the intrinsic foot muscle flaps include their relatively small size and distance of reach; therefore, preoperative planning should include alternative techniques in closure if these characteristics pose a problem intraoperatively. Complications following the use of muscle flaps in foot and ankle wound reconstruction typically involve inadequate preoperative planning and technical difficulties.[1,6]

As shown in this case report, biologic dressings for coverage over the muscle can initially be performed to preclude the need for harvesting of a large autogenous split-thickness skin graft.[8] Appropriate off-loading of the surgical site in the postoperative period is vital to flap survival, and this can be accomplished through the use of modified external fixators when traditional casts or splints do not provide adequate skeletal immobilization.[9,10] Further protection of the site with therapeutic shoe gear and regular monitoring is important for the long-term success of muscle flaps in diabetic patients.

SUMMARY

Soft tissue and skeletal reconstruction for diabetic Charcot foot wounds requires precise consideration for functional restoration of the pedal architecture to decrease the risk of reulceration, infection, and lower extremity amputation.

REFERENCES

1. Attinger CE, Ducic I, Cooper P, et al. The role of intrinsic muscle flaps of the foot for bone coverage in foot and ankle defects in diabetic and nondiabetic patients. Plast Reconstr Surg 2002;110(4):1047–54.
2. Ger R. The technique of muscle transposition and the operative treatment of traumatic and ulcerative lesions of the leg. J Trauma 1971;11:502–10.
3. Malizos KN, Gougoulias NE, Dailiana ZH, et al. Ankle and foot osteomyelitis: treatment protocol and clinical results. Injury 2010;41(3):285–93.
4. Lin SD, Chou CK, Yang CC, et al. Reconstruction of plantar heel defect using re-innervated, skin-grafted flexor digitorum brevis flap. Br J Plast Surg 1991;44(2):109–12.
5. Sakai N, Yoshida T, Okumura H. Distal plantar area reconstruction using a flexor digitorum brevis muscle flap with reverse-flow lateral plantar artery. Br J Plast Surg 2001;54(2):170–3.
6. Furukawa M, Nakagawa K, Hamada T. Long-term complications of reconstruction of the heel using a digitorum brevis muscle flap. Ann Plast Surg 1993;30(4):354–8.
7. Belczyk R, Ramanujam CL, Capobianco CM, et al. Combined midfoot arthrodesis, muscle flap coverage, and circular external fixation for the chronic ulcerated Charcot deformity. Foot Ankle Spec 2010;3(1):40–4.
8. Ramanujam CL, Zgonis T. Surgical soft tissue closure of severe diabetic foot infections: a combination of biologics, negative pressure wound therapy, and skin grafting. Clin Podiatr Med Surg 2012;29(1):143–6.
9. Clemens MW, Parikh P, Hall MM, et al. External fixators as an adjunct to wound healing. Foot Ankle Clin 2008;13(1):145–56.
10. Ramanujam CL, Facaros Z, Zgonis T. External fixation for surgical off-loading of diabetic soft tissue reconstruction. Clin Podiatr Med Surg 2011;28(1):211–6.

Total Extrusion of the Cuboid: A Case Report

John J. Stapleton, DPM[a,b,]*

KEYWORDS

• Cuboid • Extrusion • Trauma • Open wounds
• External fixation

Extensive bone defects of the midfoot and/or hindfoot as a result of trauma can be difficult to manage. In the presence of high-energy trauma, induced soft tissue injuries are also commonly encountered and further complicate the patient's surgical treatment. The incidence of total extrusion of the cuboid is rare, without any known published data or surgical guidelines. This case report describes the management of an open extruded cuboid by staged surgical interventions. Serial surgical debridements with the insertion of cemented antibiotic impregnated beads were followed by a definitive lateral column arthrodesis with the use of an autogenous structural iliac crest bone graft. Neglecting to reconstruct the lateral column of the foot will result in severe shortening and residual deformity. Arthrodesis of the lateral column with a structural bone graft is a viable option to address the shortening, instability, and severe bone loss caused by the total cuboid extrusion.

CASE REPORT

A 54-year-old man presented to the emergency room with an open foot injury after being involved in a motorcycle accident approximately 1 hour before his arrival. The patient had also sustained multiple burns throughout his body. On his arrival, the patient received intravenous (IV) fluid resuscitation, tetanus prophylaxis, and 2 g of IV cefazolin along with 160 mg of IV gentamycin. He was taken to the operating room, where he was stabilized and cleared by the trauma service of potential life-threatening injuries. The vascular status to the affected lower extremity was intact, and further intraoperative assessment of the wound revealed a 12-cm opening of the lateral portion of the foot, with complete extrusion of the cuboid and portions of the lateral cuneiform and fifth metatarsal base. The anatomic compartments of the lower extremity and foot were soft and without any evidence of compartment syndrome. The wound was thoroughly

[a] Foot and Ankle Surgery, VSAS Orthopaedics, Lehigh Valley Hospital, Cedar Crest Campus, 1250 South Cedar Crest Boulevard, Suite 110, Allentown, PA 18103, USA
[b] Penn State College of Medicine, 500 University Drive, Hershey, PA 17033, USA
* Corresponding author. Foot and Ankle Surgery, VSAS Orthopaedics, Lehigh Valley Hospital, Cedar Crest Campus, 1250 South Cedar Crest Boulevard, Suite 110, Allentown, PA 18103.
E-mail address: jostaple@hotmail.com

Clin Podiatr Med Surg 29 (2012) 327–330
doi:10.1016/j.cpm.2012.01.008   podiatric.theclinics.com
0891-8422/12/$ – see front matter © 2012 Elsevier Inc. All rights reserved.

debrided and irrigated, and an external fixator was applied to stabilize the hindfoot and ankle while spanning the lateral column of the foot to maintain anatomic length. The wound was reapproximated with a few retention sutures over a drain.

The patient was extubated postoperatively and remained hospitalized on the trauma service for pain control, local wound care, and IV antibiotics. A second irrigation and debridement of the open fracture site was performed 48 hours after the initial surgery. On this occasion the external fixator remained intact, and the wound was closed in a single-layer fashion after the insertion of cemented antibiotic impregnated beads to manage the osseous and concomitant soft tissue defect. The patient was continued on IV antibiotics, and deep vein prophylaxis was also initiated with the use of subcutaneous injections of low molecular weight heparin along with compression devices to the contralateral lower extremity.

The definitive reconstructive surgery was performed 72 hours after the second surgical debridement. On this occasion the inserted antibiotic beads were removed, and the surgical wound was again irrigated and debrided from any nonviable soft tissue. The external fixation pins were left in place, and the bar to clamp a portion of the external fixator was removed temporarily to allow access to the lateral column of the foot. Any remaining articular surfaces from the anterior process of the calcaneus, lateral portion of the navicular, and fourth metatarsal base were removed by the use of an osteotome and a curettage technique. The defect of the osseous lateral column was measured to be approximately 4.5 cm. A size-matched autogenous iliac crest bone graft (ICBG) was harvested from the ipsilateral site by the trauma service. The ICBG was then precisely fashioned and resected with a sagittal saw to match the osseous defect. A small portion of the ICBG was also resected and fashioned to reconstruct the lateral cuneiform, and was stabilized with a 3.5-mm cortical screw that was placed into the body of the navicular.

The autogenous ICBG was inlaid and stabilized provisionally with smooth wires in the lateral column. A reconstruction plate for internal fixation was bent and contoured to the lateral column, and a 3.5-mm cortical screw was placed in lag fashion across the ICBG-calcaneal interface. The plate was then tunneled proximally along the lateral aspect of the calcaneus and over the fourth metatarsal distally. The plate was secured proximally with 2 4.0-mm fully threaded cancellous screws into the calcaneus and 2 3.5-mm cortical screws into the fourth metatarsal. These screws were inserted using a percutaneous technique after tunneling of the plate. Two additional 3.5-mm cortical screws were used to stabilize the plate to the structural ICBG. The surgical wound was then closed over a drain, and the external fixator was reassembled to the preexisting half pins. The surgical drain was removed 48 hours postoperatively.

The patient continued on IV antibiotics based on fracture protocol for an additional 72 hours, at which time he was discharged from the hospital. He was instructed on pin-site care and told to keep the wound clean and dry. The surgical sutures were removed 3 weeks postoperatively. The wound healed without any signs of infection. The external fixator was removed 8 weeks after the lateral column arthrodesis. The patient was then placed into a non–weight-bearing cast for 2 weeks followed by a weight-bearing surgical boot for an additional 2 weeks. He was able to resume full ambulation with regular shoe gear at 14 weeks postoperatively, without any major complications (**Fig. 1**).

DISCUSSION

This case report describes a detailed surgical technique for the management of a total cuboid extrusion, which is rare and not commonly reported in the scientific literature.

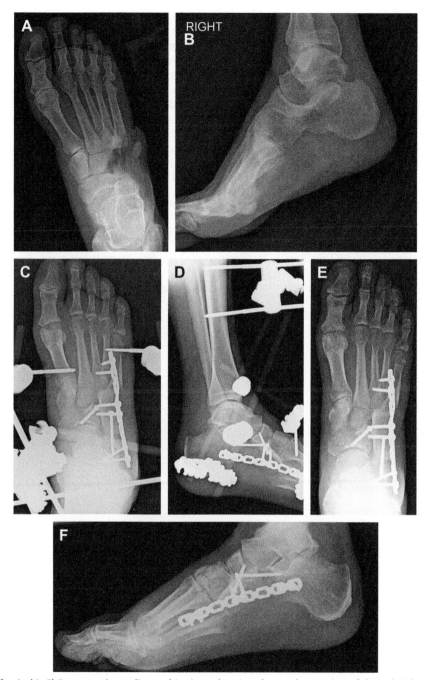

Fig. 1. (*A, B*) Preoperative radiographic views showing the total extrusion of the cuboid and the severe osseous defect at the lateral column of the foot. (*C, D*) The patient underwent serial debridements with a definitive lateral column arthrodesis, with the use of an autogenous iliac crest bone graft and combined internal and external fixation. (*E, F*) Final outcome at approximately 14 weeks postoperatively.

Other surgical alternatives to segmental traumatic bone loss include the use of bone transport, free osteocutaneous flaps, and bone grafting with external fixation.[1–3] In this case, the soft tissue envelope was amenable to primary closure without the need of a major flap coverage. Although deformity was prevented by performing a bone block arthrodesis of the lateral column, the resulting limitation of motion was evident about the midfoot and hindfoot. Anatomic alignment of the hindfoot and ankle is paramount, and a varus position of the calcaneus and/or ankle needs to be avoided. For this reason, the external fixator was used to maintain alignment of the lower extremity during the lateral column arthrodesis procedure.

In conclusion, this case report emphasizes the importance of staged reconstruction for open total extrusion of the cuboid by performing a definitive lateral column arthrodesis with the use of combined internal and external fixation.

REFERENCES

1. Facaros Z, Stapleton JJ, Polyzois V, et al. Management of foot and ankle trauma. Perioperat Nurs Clin 2011;6:35–43.
2. Memisoglu K, Hürmeydan A. Total extrusion of the talus in an adolescent: a case report. J Am Podiatr Med Assoc 2009;99:431–4.
3. Assal M, Stern R. Total extrusion of the talus. A case report. J Bone Joint Surg Am 2004;86:2726–31.

Index

Note: Page numbers of article titles are in **boldface** type.

A

Achilles tendon rupture, neglected, **291–299**
    anatomic considerations in, 291–292
    diagnosis of, 292–293
    treatment of, 293–297
Aminoglycosides
    for open fractures, 283
    for puncture wounds, 320
Amputation, for open fractures, 286
Ankle fractures, **135–186**
    anatomic considerations in, 156–157
    bimalleolar and bimalleolar equivalent, 161–162
    complications of, 180–181
    Danis-Weber
        type A, 159–161
        type B, 162–168
        type C, 171–173
    fibular
        isolated, 157–158
        proximal, 174–177
    historical review of, 156
    open, 178–179
    overview of, 155–157
    statistics on, 155–156
    surgical timing for, 179–180
    trimalleolar and trimalleolar equivalent, 168–170
Antibiotics
    for open fractures, 281–283
    for puncture wounds, 319–321
AO classification, of pilon fractures, 246
Arthrodesis
    for calcaneal fractures, 215
    for Lisfranc joint injuries, 232, 238
Arthrosis, after Lisfranc joint injuries, 241
Avascular necrosis, in talar neck fractures, 190–191, 200

B

Berndt and Harty classification, of talar dome fractures, 195
Bimalleolar and bimalleolar equivalent fractures, 161–162
Blisters, in calcaneal fractures, 208

Clin Podiatr Med Surg 29 (2012) 331–339
doi:10.1016/S0891-8422(12)00035-3
0891-8422/12/$ – see front matter © 2012 Elsevier Inc. All rights reserved.

podiatric.theclinics.com

Bohler classification, of calcaneal fractures, 206
Bone grafts
    for calcaneal fractures, 215
    for cuboid extrusion, **327–330**
    for open fractures, 286
Bracing, for Achilles tendon rupture, 294

C

Calcaneal fractures, **205–220**
    anatomic considerations in, 205–206
    challenges for, 206–209
    injuries associated with, 206–209
    prevalence of, 205
    radiography for, 206
    treatment of
        approaches to, 209–215
        bone grafting in, 215
        closure assistance in, 215–216
        complications of, 216–217
Calcaneal gait, in Achilles tendon rupture, 294
Calcaneoplasty, for calcaneal fractures, 214–215
Catheterization, compartment, 305
Cedell fractures, 199–200
Cefoperazone, for puncture wounds, 320
Ceftazidime, for puncture wounds, 320
Cephalosporins
    for open fractures, 283
    for puncture wounds, 320
Cerclage wire fixation, for ankle fractures
    Danis-Weber type B, 166
    Danis-Weber type C, 173
Charcot foot, intrinsic muscle flaps for, **323–326**
Ciprofloxacin
    for open fractures, 283
    for puncture wounds, 319–320
Circular ring fixation, for calcaneal fractures, 213
Closed reduction
    for calcaneal fractures, 210
    for Lisfranc joint injuries, 230
    for pilon fractures, 253
Compartment syndrome, **301–310**
    anatomy of, 302–304
    case studies of, 307–308
    catheterization in, 305
    chronic exertional, 301–302, 306
    clinical presentation of, 304
    diagnosis of, 301
    in calcaneal fractures, 208–209
    in Lisfranc joint injuries, 238–240
    in pilon fractures, 249

incidence of, 301
pathophysiology of, 302
surgical treatment of, 305–307
Compression screw fixation, for Lisfranc joint injuries, 233
Computed tomography
for Lisfranc joint injuries, 226
for pilon fractures, 252–253
for puncture wounds, 316, 318
Coonrad-Bugg trap, 162
Cotton test, 176
Cuboid, total extrusion of, **327–330**

D

Danis-Weber classification, of ankle fractures, 157
type A, 159–161
type B, 162–168
type C, 171–173
Débridement
for ankle fractures, 178
for cuboid extrusion, **327–330**
for open fractures, 283–284
for puncture wounds, 319–320
Degenerative joint disease, after ankle fractures, 180–181
Delayed union
of ankle fractures, 180–181
of calcaneal fractures, 217
Delta frame fixation, for calcaneal fractures, 213–214
Deltoid ligament rupture, in ankle fractures, 161–162
Destot classification, of pilon fractures, 246
Diabetic foot
intrinsic muscle flaps for, **323–326**
puncture wounds in, 313–314

E

Endoscopic fasciotomy, for compartment syndrome, 307
Essex-Lopresti classification, of calcaneal fractures, 206
Extended lateral approach, to calcaneal fractures, 211
External fixation
for calcaneal fractures, 213–214
for cuboid extrusion, **327–330**
for Lisfranc joint injuries, 232–233
for open fractures, 285
for pilon fractures, 249–250, 256–267
for talar fractures, 192

F

Fascial advancement, for neglected Achilles tendon rupture, 295
Fasciotomy, for compartment syndrome, 209, 305–307

Fibular fractures
  isolated, 157–158
  proximal, 174–177
  with tibial fractures, 248
Fleck sign, in Lisfranc joint injuries, 225–226, 228
Flexor digitorum brevis muscle flap, for diabetic Charcot foot, **323–326**
Flexor digitorum longus tendon transfer, for neglected Achilles tendon rupture, 295
Flexor hallucis tendon transfer, for neglected Achilles tendon rupture, 295–297
Foreign bodies, in puncture wounds, 313–314, 316–319
Fortin classification, of talar body fractures, 194
Fracture(s)
  ankle, **135–186**
  calcaneal, **205–220**
  open, **279–290**
    ankle, 178–179
    talar, 193
  pilon, **243–278**
  talar, **187–203**
Fracture blisters, in calcaneal fractures, 208

G

Gastrocnemius recession, for neglected Achilles tendon rupture, 295
Gaweda classification, of Lisfranc joint injuries, 225
Gentamicin
  for open fractures, 283
  for puncture wounds, 320
Grafts, for open fractures, 286
Gustilio and Anderson classification, of open fracture, 280–281
Gustilio principles, for open fractures, 280

H

Hardcastle classification, of Lisfranc joint injuries, 224–225
Hardware removal, after calcaneal fractures, 217
Hawkins classification, of talar fractures
  lateral process, 198
  neck, 190
Henderson classification, of ankle fractures, 157

I

Immobilization
  for ankle fractures, 159–160
  for Lisfranc joint injuries, 229–230
  for open fractures, 285
  for puncture wounds, 321
  for talar fractures, 189
    body, 197
    lateral process, 198
    neck, 191–192
    posterior process, 200

Infections
    after calcaneal fractures, 216
    after open fractures, 281–283
    after pilon fractures, 268–269
    of puncture wounds, 320–321
Interfragmentary screw fixation, for ankle fractures, 163–165
Internal fixation, open reduction with. *See* Open reduction and internal fixation.
Intramedullary screw fixation, for ankle fractures, 159–160
Irrigation
    for cuboid extrusion, **327–330**
    for open fractures, 284
    for puncture wounds, 319–320

K

Krakow stitch, for neglected Achilles tendon rupture, 294–295

L

Lateral process fractures, talar, 197–198
Lisfranc joint injuries, **221–242**
    anatomic considerations in, 221–223
    classifications of, 224–225
    complications of, 238–240
    diagnosis of, 225–227
    historical review of, 221
    mechanism of, 223–224
    postoperative course in, 237–238
    prevalence of, 221
    treatment of, 227–238
Locking screw fixation, for ankle fractures, 164

M

Magnetic resonance imaging
    for Achilles tendon rupture, 293
    for Lisfranc joint injuries, 226
Maisonneuve fractures, 174–177
Malleolar fractures. *See* Ankle fractures.
Malunion, of calcaneal fractures, 217
Mangled Extremity Severity Score, for open fractures, 286–287
Myerson classification, of Lisfranc joint injuries, 225
Myotendinous lengthening, for neglected Achilles tendon rupture, 295

N

National Research Council classification, of open fractures, 280
Negative wound therapy
    for calcaneal fractures, 215–216
    for pilon fractures, 268

Nonunion
    of ankle fractures, 180–181
    of calcaneal fractures, 217
    of pilon fractures, 268

O

Open fractures, **279–290**
    ankle, 178–179
    classifications of, 280–281
    evaluation of, 279–280
    incidence of, 279
    infection protocols for, 281–283
    talar, 193
    treatment of
        amputation as, 286
        closure in, 285–286
        complications of, 286–287
        debridement in, 283–284
        fixation in, 284–285
        goals of, 279–280
        irrigation in, 284
Open reduction and internal fixation
    for ankle fractures, 178–179
    for calcaneal fractures, 210–214
    for lateral process talar fractures, 198
    for Lisfranc joint injuries, 230, 232–237
    for open fractures, 284–285
    for pilon fractures, 254–267
    for talar fractures, 189
        body, 197
        neck, 192
Orthosis, for Achilles tendon rupture, 294
Osteoarthritis
    after ankle fractures, 180–181
    after talar fractures, 200
Osteochondral talar fractures, 194–195
Osteochondritis dissecans, 194–195
Osteomyelitis, in puncture wounds, 314, 320

P

Pain, in compartment syndrome, 304
Penicillin(s), for puncture wounds, 320
Penicillin G, for open fractures, 283
Percutaneous approach, to calcaneal fracture repair, 210
Pilon fractures, **243–278**
    anatomic considerations in, 247–249
    classification of, 246–247
    description of, 247–248
    incidence of, 243

injuries associated with, 249
mechanism of injury in, 243–244
overview of, 247–249
treatment of
    closed reduction, 253
    complications of, 268–273
    conservative, 249
    controversy about, 245–246
    external fixation, 256–257
    open methods for, 254–256
    planning for, 249–253
    postoperative care in, 268–273
    preferred method (staged external and internal fixation), 257–268
    skeletal traction, 254
Pin fixation
    for Lisfranc joint injuries, 230
    for open fractures, 285
    for talar fractures, 189
Piperacillin, for puncture wounds, 320
Plate fixation
    for ankle fractures, 164–167, 173
    for calcaneal fractures, 210–211
Posterior process fractures, talar, 199–200
Pressure measurement, in compartment syndrome, 305
Pseudomonas aeruginosa, in puncture wounds, 318
Puncture wounds, **311–322**
    causes of, 311–314
    complications of, 311–312
    epidemiology of, 311–314
    evaluation of, 315–316
    imaging of, 316–318
    in diabetic foot, 313–314
    microbiology of, 312–313, 318
    presentation of, 314
    treatment of
        infected, 320–321
        uninfected, 318–320

Q

Quenu and Kuss classification, of Lisfranc joint injuries, 224

R

Radiography
    for calcaneal fractures, 206
    for Lisfranc joint injuries, 225–226, 228
    for puncture wounds, 316, 318
    for talar fractures, 189
Recession techniques, for neglected Achilles tendon rupture, 295
Ring fixation, for calcaneal fractures, 213

Rowe classification, of calcaneal fractures, 206
Ruedi and Allgower classification, of pilon fractures, 246–247

S

Saline irrigation, for open fractures, 284
Sanders classification, of calcaneal fractures, 206
Screw fixation
 for ankle fractures
  Danis-Weber type A, 159–160
  Danis-Weber type B, 163–167
  Danis-Weber type C, 171–173
  proximal fibular, 175–177
  trimalleolar, 169–170
 for calcaneal fractures, 210
 for Lisfranc joint injuries, 230, 232–233, 238
 for talar fractures, 189
Sensory deficits, in compartment syndrome, 304
Shepherd fractures, 199–200
Sinus tarsi approach, to calcaneal fractures, 211–213
Skeletal traction, for pilon fractures, 249, 254
Skin grafts, for open fractures, 286
Sneppen classification, of talar body fractures, 194
Soap irrigation, for open fractures, 284
Steinmann pin fixation, for calcaneal fractures, 213
Syndesmotic complex, injury of, 174–177

T

Talar fractures, **187–203**
 anatomic considerations in, 187–188
 body, 193–197
 complications of, 200
 evaluation of, 188–189
 head, 189
 incidence of, 187
 lateral process, 197–198
 neck, 189–193
 osteochondral, 194–195
 posterior process, 199–200
Tarsometatarsal joint injuries. *See* Lisfranc joint injuries.
Tendon transfers, for neglected Achilles tendon rupture, 295–296
Tension band wiring, for ankle fractures, 164
Tetanus immunization
 for open fractures, 280
 for puncture wounds, 318–319
Tibial fractures, pilon. *See* Pilon fractures.
Ticarcillin, for puncture wounds, 320
TightRope device, for ankle fractures, 175–177
Trauma. *See also* Fracture(s).
 Achilles tendon rupture, **291–299**
 compartment syndrome in. *See* Compartment syndrome.

cuboid extrusion, **327–330**
Lisfranc joint, **221–242**
puncture wounds, **311–322**
Trimalleolar and trimalleolar equivalent fractures, 168–170
Tscherne soft tissue classification system, 247

U

Ultrasonography, for puncture wounds, 316, 318

V

Vacuum-assisted closure, for open fractures, 286
V-Y lengthening, for neglected Achilles tendon rupture, 295

W

Weber clamp, for Lisfranc joint injuries, 231
Wire fixation
    for ankle fractures, 164, 166
    for Lisfranc joint injuries, 230–231, 235–236
    for talar fractures, 189
Wound(s), puncture. *See* Puncture wounds.
Wound closure, for open fractures, 285–286

Z

ZipTight device, for ankle fractures, 175–177, 181

Moving?

Make sure your subscription moves with you!

To notify us of your new address, find your **Clinics Account Number** (located on your mailing label above your name), and contact customer service at:

Email: journalscustomerservice-usa@elsevier.com

800-654-2452 (subscribers in the U.S. & Canada)
314-447-8871 (subscribers outside of the U.S. & Canada)

Fax number: 314-447-8029

Elsevier Health Sciences Division
Subscription Customer Service
3251 Riverport Lane
Maryland Heights, MO 63043

*To ensure uninterrupted delivery of your subscription, please notify us at least 4 weeks in advance of move.

Printed and bound by CPI Group (UK) Ltd, Croydon, CR0 4YY

03/10/2024

01040456-0017